ALZHEIMER'S
A TO Z

A Quick-Reference Guide

JYTTE LOKVIG, MA • JOHN D. BECKER, MD

New Harbinger Publications, Inc.

Publisher's Note

Care has been taken to confirm the accuracy of the information presented and to describe generally accepted practices. However, the authors, editors, and publisher are not responsible for errors or omissions or for any consequences from application of the information in this book and make no warranty, express or implied, with respect to the contents of the publication.

The authors, editors, and publisher have exerted every effort to ensure that any drug selection and dosage set forth in this text are in accordance with current recommendations and practice at the time of publication. However, in view of ongoing research, changes in government regulations, and the constant flow of information relating to drug therapy and drug reactions, the reader is urged to check the package insert for each drug for any change in indications and dosage and for added warnings and precautions. This is particularly important when the recommended agent is a new or infrequently employed drug.

Some drugs and medical devices presented in this publication may have Food and Drug Administration (FDA) clearance for limited use in restricted research settings. It is the responsibility of the health care provider to ascertain the FDA status of each drug or device planned for use in their clinical practice.

Distributed in Canada by Raincoast Books

Copyright © 2004 by Jytte Lokvig and John Becker
New Harbinger Publications, Inc.
5674 Shattuck Avenue
Oakland, CA 94609

Cover design by Amy Shoup
Cover image by Rubberball/Photography/Veer
Edited by Kayla Sussell
Acquired by Spencer Smith
Text design by Michele Waters-Kermes

ISBN-10 1-57224-395-3
ISBN-13 978-1-57224-395-8

Printed in the United States of America

New Harbinger Publications' Web site address: www.newharbinger.com

09   08   07

10   9   8   7   6   5   4   3   2

Read one section a day, and in no time at all, you'll have a deeper understanding of Alzheimer's. Instead of asking, "why didn't I think of that?" you'll learn positive and creative approaches to caring for your loved one.

> —Brenda Avadian, MA, author of *Where's My Shoes? My Father's Walk Through Alzheimer's* and *Finding the Joy in Alzheimer's*

This book belongs in the library of everyone involved with the care of someone with Alzheimer's. Rich with examples of how to handle even the most challenging situations, the information is easy to access and understand and the approach to care is compassionate and insightful.

> —Jacqueline Marcell, author of *Elder Rage, or Take My Father... Please! How to Survive Caring for Aging Parents*

In light of the rapidly expanding proportion of elderly in our population, Alzheimer's disease looms as the single greatest health-related problem facing the United States. The emotional burden on family, friends, and caregivers is already immeasurable and will only get worse in coming years. This book is a treasure trove of sage advice and valuable tips for every imaginable situation one might encounter in caring for an Alzheimer's patient. Lokvig is to be heartily congratulated for a job well done.

> —Rudolph E. Tanzi, Ph.D., professor of neurology at Harvard Medical School and director of the Genetic and Aging Research Unit at Massachusetts General Hospital

Dedicated to my parents, whose lives were examples of creativity, joy, and service—and to my dear friend Bahtee Ames, without whom this book would never have happened.

—Jytte Lokvig

I dedicate this book to my father who had alzheimer's and to my mother who cared for him as long as she was able.

—John D. Becker

Contents

Foreword

Alzheimer's disease is one of the leading causes of misery in older individuals and their families. Medical intervention and drug treatment are often required when thinking, reasoning, and memory begin to fade, and when screaming, wandering, and sleeplessness begin. As the disease progresses, paranoid thinking and depression are not unusual

It is true, however, that great strides have been made in the scientific understanding of Alzheimer's disease. Although the cause is still unknown, a possible genetic basis for some forms of the disease is rapidly becoming clearer. Changes in brain chemistry are also becoming better understood. These discoveries are heralded in frequent headlines in the news media proclaiming another step forward in unraveling the mystery of Alzheimer's disease.

Society may applaud the scientific achievements, but these advances do not address the emotional, physical, and financial toll that the disorder exacts from the personal lives of afflicted individuals and their families. The simplest activities of daily living become progressively more difficult and eventually impossible. Emotional connections become so eroded and faint that family members are never quite sure whether the afflicted Alzheimer's patient knows who they are, or even whether they are present. It is the worst of all possible conditions: a chronic illness that robs people of their most human feature, the ability to think and reason, and deprives family members of a loved one who remains physiologically alive but is emotionally no longer present.

Those who are familiar with the disorder know that as the disease progresses, attention must be directed toward family members and caregivers who invariably need a great deal of support. Caring for someone afflicted with Alzheimer's is very difficult and often thankless labor. It is hard work and often demoralizing to care for an Alzheimer's disease patient. Any useful advice that will help in caring for these patients is precious indeed.

Alzheimer's A to Z by Jytte Lokvig answers this need: it is filled with practical suggestions for family members and caregivers alike. Written by an experienced caregiver herself, there is great clinical wisdom and experience packed into a most readable format. This book should be read by all who care for the Alzheimer's disease patient. My hope is that medical professionals will also read this book in order to gain a greater appreciation of the day-to-day problems associated with taking care of an Alzheimer's patient that might not be readily apparent in an office visit or a nursing home consultation. Everyone who is concerned about this terrible disorder will find comfort and wisdom along with very practical advice in this accessible, clearly written book.

—Carl Salzman, MD, Professor of
Psychiatry, Harvard Medical School

Preface

Several years ago, a friend asked me help out with her mother while she was away on an extended business trip. Her mother had Alzheimer's and needed someone to visit with her for a few hours a day. I had read about Alzheimer's, of course, but had never met anyone with the disease. I had no idea what to expect.

My first visit was a disaster. My new acquaintance greeted me sweetly enough, but she spent the entire visit worrying about who I was and what I was doing there. None of my attempts at conversation worked and I left feeling a complete failure. Determined to make this work, on my next visit, I decided to share my interests with her and take her to one of my favorite art galleries. She was engrossed.

From then on we visited galleries together regularly and began making collages from the gallery announcements that we'd picked up along the way. It wasn't long before she was creating collages on her own. And while she cut and pasted, we talked. We talked about our lives, loves, funny experiences, and some sad ones. Her stories were often disjointed and confused, but over time I pieced together a picture of her life. We became true friends. Other families started coming to me for help and soon we were a whole group. We made music and art, wrote stories, and discussed everything under the sun. We visited the library and museums, went to the movies, and picnicked by the river.

I read everything I could find on Alzheimer's disease, but there was very little that helped me with my daily situations, so I had to find my own solutions. A person with Alzheimer's disease or dementia is not "sick" as such, but rather is in an altered state of mind and is still capable of having a rich life. It soon became clear to me that my friends all thought of themselves as quite normal in a world that felt increasingly confusing to them.

I address the "normal" in everyone and work with their individual interests and needs. Together we invent the days as we go along. The goal is to have rich and fulfilling experiences, no matter how insignificant they might appear to others. The most special times occur when we just talk. I mostly listen, because everyone needs an ear. I work with folks from diverse backgrounds, with different interests, temperaments, and all levels of dementia. I've found that certain attitudes, ways of communication, and approaches are consistently effective with everyone, regardless of the degree of impairment.

Over the years I've shared these tools with families and care facilities with most satisfying results. I decided it was time to share them with you. This book is compiled from my own experiences and the situations that invariably come up for other caregivers.

John Becker, MD, has taken time out from his busy practive to review, add to, and scrutinize the medical information in this book. He has always impressed me with his knowledge of the special needs of the elderly, particularly those with dementia and alzheimer's.

May this book be of use to you.

—Jytte Lokvig

Acknowledgments

This book is a labor of love that could not have happened without my many friends with Alzheimer's disease, who over the years have taught me how to appreciate the smallest pleasures found in every new day. My gratitude also to the many families who have so generously shared their own experiences.

Many persons contributed to this project and it's hard to single out any one. For several years my family and friends stood by me and supported my single-minded obsession while I was working on this book.

Special appreciation goes to several professionals who generously have shared their expertise. First of all, very special thanks to John Becker, MD, for his input and scrutiny of the sections on Alzheimer's and health. Teresa A. Holzer, DDS, advised on dental health; Mahlon R. Soloway, MD, advised on eye health. Edward Williams, DPM, advised on foot care, and Dr. Wendy Anita Van Dilla, naturopathic physician, advised on alternative remedies; Shannon Broderick Bulman, Attorney, advised on legal issues. Also thanks to the staff of the Ombudsman's program, the Agency on Aging for the State of New Mexico, and the Alzheimer's Association for their input and consistent support and advice.

Rockne Tarkington, screenwriter, suggested using "scenes" and dialogue, which gave me the key to the user-friendly format I was seeking. Damaris Ames has been one of my strongest supporters from day one. Deanna Bellinger, director of NAMI (National Association of the Mentally Impaired), in Southeastern Arizona, generously shared her experiences with me. My friend Cecelia Davidson, artist, is my most discriminating reader; my friend Douglas Houston is my irreplaceable computer guru. Thank you to Ruth Dennis, Alzheimer's activities director, and Catherine Wallace, Director of Marian House Alzheimer's Home in Sydney, Australia for sharing their innovative ideas with me.

And many thanks to my editors at New Harbinger, Spencer Smith and Kayla Sussell. Working with them was a pleasure.

Introduction

Taking care of a person with Alzheimer's is a difficult and demanding task. This book was written to help you deal with many of the situations that you're likely to encounter as a caregiver. Typical problems based on actual events and effective solutions are arranged in alphabetical order. You can read the book from beginning to end or you can choose to go directly to a specific problem. At the end of each segment you'll find referrals to other relevant topics.

The situations we describe may not be identical to yours, but they're likely to be similar enough for you to adapt them to your needs. We frequently refer to "Mom" and "Dad," although, in fact, you may be caring for another relative, friend, partner, or client. We haven't tried to distinguish between the different stages of the disease because we've found that, in all cases, the most important factors are attitude and communication.

As the disease progresses, the person's mental scope may become narrower because of diminished capacity and perception, but their emotional needs don't change. Effective caregiving involves creative approaches to maintaining dignity, and a sense of trust. If this information is new to you, some of our ideas may sound unorthodox, but as you put them into practice, you'll find that they make sense.

It used to be thought that a caregiver should constantly reinforce "reality" with a demented person. However, because Alzheimer's disease actually destroys the brain cells responsible for short-term memory, "reality therapy" is futile. We now understand that validation of a person's feelings and thoughts is, in fact, the most important thing we can do for eachother, no matter what our mental state might be. With an Alzheimer's person this sometimes means using white (or "loving") lies.

Alzheimer's disease causes memory loss. People with dementia may not be able to remember what happened in the previous hour, whereas they may have perfect recall of an event from their child-hood. As the present becomes increasingly confusing to them, Alzheimer's patients often retreat into their past. When we first encounter this in a loved one, it's our instinct to do everything in our power to bring the person back to the present. However, when this happens, it's important for us to realize that he or she may actually be reliving rather than merely remembering an event, and to help that person get back to the present, we're more effective when we validate his or her experience by reacting as though we're sharing it.

You may have qualms about telling white lies. But, in this case, your response should be based on the Alzheimer's person's reality at the moment. Your lie is in fact their truth and it is the kindest and most considerate thing you can do for them. For example, suppose you've opened your heart and home to your mother since she was diagnosed with Alzheimer's and became unable to live by herself any longer. She may be very angry at being uprooted from her own home, and may be so resistant to your care that you've seriously considered placing her in a care facility, even if it means mortgaging your own house to pay for it.

Before you take such a drastic step, consider reading through this book and using our suggestions to explore new avenues to reach your mother and to help her through this. She may not be able to express her feelings to you anymore, and she's most likely afraid and confused. Her whole world has been turned upside down and often she has no idea where she is or who she is. If she lashes out at you in anger, she's probably trying to let you know just how frightened she really is. She needs you to be strong, calm, and reassuring.

In the beginning, you'll have to learn to ignore her outbursts and reassure her that you love and appreciate her. The first few weeks will be the most difficult, but with practice, your helpful reactions will become second nature. It's by no means an easy path, but instead of mourning the loss of your mother as she used to be, celebrate the person she is now, a vital human being who still has a lot of love, laughter, and enjoyment left to share with you.

A

Acceptance

Dad's so different now from what he was like just a few years ago, before the onset of his dementia. It's been very hard for you to accept the truth that the father you once knew will never return. Sometimes, when he says or does something familiar and behaves just like his old self, you want to hang onto him to keep him from disappearing again. It's natural to grieve your loss, but at the same time, for the sake of your own emotional survival, try to learn to accept him as he is. He often lives in an altered reality. Try to go into this space with him and see things from his point of view. This isn't easy and it will take some time for you to get used to doing it, but the payoff will be a much smoother relationship with him.

Although it's a fact that your father's dementia is not likely to improve, he still can be a meaningful person in your life. Take your caregiving experience one day at a time and set reasonable goals for yourself. Appreciate small achievements like an easy bath time or a pleasant outing. And when you make it through a whole day without a hitch, celebrate your successes.

Don't be too hard on yourself, because the process of acceptance takes time. Even though your father's not the same anymore, who he is now can still be interesting, fun, and even lovable. Don't beat yourself up when you feel sadness or grief coming over you. Instead, ask your father for a big hug and give him one in return.

Your mother may mistake you for her sister or even her mother but it's obvious that she recognizes you as someone she trusts and loves. Your willingness to be accepted as these other important people from her life will give you the opportunity to learn more about her, not only who she was as your mother, but who she is as a human being.

You've thought of Mom as your best friend for most of your adult life, so when she needed it, it seemed only natural to take her into your home to care for her. Now that you've accustomed yourself to the slower pace of her life, all in all, things are going well. But there may come a day you'll wake her for breakfast and she'll behave as if she has never met you before. She may clutch her blanket in obvious fear and scream at you as a "stranger" who has invaded her bedroom. She may accuse you of keeping her prisoner and not allowing her to go back to her own home. You can explain until you're blue in the face why she's living with you now, but she will sulk and be unresponsive to your pleas until you're overwhelmed with sadness and guilt. You'll try to comfort her but she'll keep pulling away from you in her panic. You'll feel as though your heart is breaking. Your own mother won't know who you are and you won't have any idea about what to do.

It may take you some time to collect your thoughts and build up your nerve to try again. But when you hesitantly open her door she may be sitting on the edge of her bed, humming to herself. When she sees you, her face may beam loving recognition as she says to you, "Hi Sis."

(*See also:* Alzheimer's Disease; Comprehension; Dementia; Empathy; Normal; Reality; Validation)

■ ■ ■ ■ ■ ■ ■ ■

Activities

Activities are essential for the mental well-being of everyone, and your uncle Richard's no exception. He may not be able to recall many of the things you do together, but the experiences still help him feel enriched and involved. As a successful caregiver, you'll discover a healthy balance between maintenance, such as showers and meals, and activities that he does both by himself and with you that will provide pleasure and personal fulfillment.

Retirement has been difficult for Uncle Richard. He no longer has his job to give him a reason to get up in the morning, and he misses the sense of validation he felt from receiving a paycheck.

Successful retirees find substitute activities to keep themselves stimulated and vital, but because of his dementia, Uncle Richard is not able to do this for himself. He needs you to help make things happen for him. In the beginning it may take some extra effort on your part, but soon the result will be a happier man and an easier life for both of you. This book has many ideas for games, group projects, excursions, and special activity areas at home.

The success of Uncle Richard's projects depends a lot on your demeanor. However uncomplicated the project might be, it's your attitude that will give it legitimacy and importance. No matter what his activity is, it's important for you to take it seriously. For example, suppose that Uncle Richard's been restless since he finished breakfast. He needs something to do to help him get back to feeling good about himself. What can you do to help him?

Begin by asking for his help. For example, you could say, "Excuse me, Uncle Richard, are you busy right now? I sure could use your help with this. May I show you? See this stack of catalogs? They're all mixed up. Could you help me sort them out, please? You've always been so good at that sort of thing."

After he agrees, go through the catalogs and say something like, "Let's see . . . several gardening catalogs, gourmet catalogs, furniture catalogs, and Avon catalogs are all mixed up in this huge pile . . . can you make heads or tails of them?"

Encourage him to approach this task in any way he chooses. He may decide to spend all his time looking at only one catalog or he may restack them. Whatever he does, thank him for his help. It takes a lot of patience on your part, but in the process you are letting him know that you value his help and, in turn, you're affirming his feeling of self-determination. It's important that you do not talk to him as if he were a child; he's demented but he's not stupid.

(See also: Exercise; Games; Kitchen; Outings; Personal Space; Projects; Reading; Singing)

Activities

A ■■■■■■■
Affection

Your cousin Al has a lot of trouble with his speech these days, so you're relying more and more on nonverbal communication. You've discovered that affectionate gestures like hugs, kisses, and hand-holding seem to calm Al down and make him more responsive to you. You make a point of touching and hugging him many times a day, but it's also important that, occasionally, you ask for his permission. For example, you could say, "Al, may I have a hug from you, please?" He will be likely to beam as he straightens his back and reaches out to hold you. For one brief moment you may feel as if you're six years old again, and he's your big, strong cousin, who never lets anything bad happen to you. You feel it and he feels it. And after the hug, you can say to him, "Thank you, your hugs always make me feel so good." Or try asking, "May I give you a back rub?"

By asking for Al's consent, you're offering him a choice that helps to boost his feeling of control over his life. He may surprise you by becoming much more cooperative and attentive.

(*See also:* Massage; Questions)

■■■■■■■
Age

Since growing old doesn't fit very comfortably with our youth-conscious society, age can be a touchy subject once we reach our forties or fifties. Aging is hard on everyone, so why should anyone presume it's okay to exclaim to an elderly person, "You're ninety, wow! How does it feel?" when we wouldn't dream of exclaiming, "You're fifty-five, wow! How does it feel?"

Your mother often becomes upset if people around her make a big deal about her "ripe old age," so you may have to intercede on her behalf. Others may talk to you about her in her presence as if she can't understand a word they say. But that's not so. She can understand quite a lot, and the subject of her age may come up often. She probably doesn't remember her actual age, but she may still relate being in her eighties or nineties as being "very old." That can be a depressing thought.

So, instead of dwelling on her age, try to encourage a conversation about how old everyone feels inside, "in spirit." In discussions like these, your Mom is likely to recall the events of her young adulthood or college days, which may have been the times in her life when she felt the most independent and empowered.

(*See also:* Birthdays; Comprehension; Dignity; Empathy; Normal)

■ ■ ■ ■ ■ ■ ■ ■

Aggression

Suppose one day your Grandma suddenly lashes out, kicking you and screaming incoherently. Clearly, something triggered her outburst. But before you can deal with anything else, you'll need to calm her down. In a firm but gentle voice, and loudly enough to grab her attention, you could say, "Grandma, I can't understand what you're saying. Please lower your voice so I can hear you. I want to help you." Or, you could say very loudly, "Grandma, *I love you!*"

Then, if she seems receptive, you could say, "May I have a hug? I need a hug from you, please." Put your arms around her and hold her gently but firmly until you feel the tension leave her body. Once she's calmer, change her environment by taking her into another room. As you help her to sit down, say, "Grandma, I love you and it hurts me to see you this upset. I want to help you. Can you tell me what's happening?"

She might respond with something like, "I want to go home. You're keeping me prisoner here! I don't want to be here. I want to go home!" She may be talking about the small apartment she lived in before she came to live with you. Or she might mean her childhood home. Regardless, it will serve no useful purpose while she is in her current state of mind to remind her that her "home" is now occupied by someone else. At other times, she seems to understand and accept this fact, but probably not now. You could say to her, "Maybe we can go later, Grandma, but I'm about to fix lunch, and you told me a few minutes ago that you were starved, so why don't we eat lunch first?"

You have a leisurely lunch and after you've finished, you might say, "Have I told you lately how glad I am that we're able to spend so much time together? I'm so happy that you're in my life!"

IN PUBLIC

Suppose you and Grandma have just had a delightful lunch at a nice restaurant, and now it's time to go home. You exit the restaurant and try to steer her through the mass of people on the crowded sidewalk. Suddenly something spooks her. She yanks her arm away and tries to loosen your grip as she screams, "Help, call the police! Call the police! Help me, I'm being kidnapped!"

You're astounded as she pummels your arm with all her might, because you had no idea she is that strong. Some people stop and stare. Others quickly look away, not wanting to get involved. One man steps up to "help." Grandma grabs his arm and falls into his embrace, giving you no choice but to release her. As you look into the man's face, you're startled to see that he's glaring at you!

This is as upsetting as anything that has happened so far. Thoughts of nursing homes and restraints are taking shape in the back of your mind, and these ideas look mighty good to you right now. To strangers, Grandma looks like a perfectly lucid, normal woman, while you're so upset you probably look like the wacky one. This man thinks you are a *bad* person. You're mortified.

Take a deep breath and don't speak until you can use a normal tone of voice, then calmly turn to the stranger and say, "Thanks so much for helping me with my grandmother. It can get pretty difficult for her in crowds like this because her Alzheimer's sometimes makes her claustrophobic. I appreciate your concern."

For once you actually might need to speak to Grandma in a patronizing tone to get your point across to the "rescuer." Unfortunately, most people assume that's the way caregivers are supposed to communicate. Say to her, "Grandma, we need to go home now. Be a dear and say thank you to the nice man."

Once you're finally away from the crowd, the real challenge is to not be angry with her. Most likely she will have already forgotten the incident. However, for your own sanity, you may need to get it off your chest, so call someone from your Alzheimer's support group, a

Aggression

good friend, or a family member so you can share your experiences and feelings.

You and your mother are browsing at a department store, when a salesperson notices a bruise on her arm and makes a comment about it. Suppose Mom's immediate reaction is to exclaim loudly, "My daughter did that! She beats me and she locks me up! Hurry up, call the police!"

While the salesperson is trying to regain her composure, you grab Mom by the hand and head for your car. Safely at home, you forget about the incident until a police officer and someone from Adult Protective Services appear at your door. Yikes! It takes a lot of phone calls and explanations to convince the two of them that your mother has Alzheimer's disease and the mark on her arm is a harmless bruise. They finally leave you with wishes of good luck. You don't ever want to go through that again, so what should you do?

You can understand why the salesperson called the authorities; after all, your mother looks normal and can sound totally lucid. The next time something like this happens, don't leave without an explanation. Having Mom wear a medical alert bracelet engraved with "Alzheimer's" or "memory-impaired" will convey her condition to others instantly. You can also contact your local law enforcement agency and any emergency rooms in your area. Give them your mother's picture and physical description. If a situation like this happens again, ask the other person involved to call the police department to confirm your mother's illness. That way you'll avoid all the stressful follow-up events.

(*See also:* Conversations; Diversions; Empathy; Going Home; Identification; Safe Return)

■ ■ ■ ■ ■ ■ ■ ■

Agitation

You were very apprehensive about moving your brother into your spare room, but now that he's lived with you for some time, it's been fine. He's been easygoing and you've enjoyed his company far more than you'd expected. Lately, however, he's been completely different. He's angry, short-tempered, and uncooperative. He'll lash out at you one minute and withdraw into despondency the next. You've tried many of the suggestions you found in this book, but nothing seems to help. It's been difficult and confusing for you. It's possible there's a good cause for your brother's feelings that has nothing to do with you. Consider consulting his doctor if you suspect that his problem might be physical. Look over the following list and if the answer to any of these questions is yes, that might be the cause for the change in your brother's behavior:

> Has his physical condition changed lately? For example, is he experiencing constipation, dental problems, or dehydration?

> Is he reacting to medications?

> Was anything changed in his room recently?

> Are his shoes too tight? Do his clothes bother him?

> If he's wearing a brief (an adult diaper) or a pad, is it uncomfortable or wet?

> Have you noticed a sudden decline in his comprehension or speech? (Note that he may be aware of this and may need extra support from you.)

> Has his hearing or sight changed lately?

(*See also:* Aggression; Body Language; Depression; Diversions; Environment; Health)

■ ■ ■ ■ ■ ■ ■ ■
Alternative Remedies

Consult your physician before using any medicine, including any alternative or complementary medicines. Today, many doctors support alternative healing methods. However, if your doctor is not comfortable with these remedies, you may want to consult a holistic health provider. You already may be using some of the following substances with your daily vitamin supplement. As much as possible, you'll want to incorporate these substances into a daily diet or a smoothie (Vukovic 1998).

Aloe Vera is a wonderful healing agent for burns. (Aloe is an attractive and easy-to-cultivate house or garden plant. You can break off a leaf when you need it.)

Arnica gel soothes strains and aching muscles (for external use only).

Bilberry may be one of the few substances that can halt macular degeneration of the eye. It is also helpful with night blindness and cataracts. It acts as a diuretic and urinary tract antiseptic.

Coenzyme Q$_{10}$ is a vitamin-like substance found naturally in the body, but it declines as we age. It is a potent antioxidant with effects resembling those of vitamin E, only more powerful. It's been prescribed for years in Japan for millions of people with heart disease. Coenzyme Q$_{10}$ is a strong immune-system booster especially beneficial for circulation and tissue oxygenation, and is critical to cell growth. It's also used to treat mental dysfunctions such as schizophrenia and Alzheimer's disease. Coenzyme Q$_{10}$ is oil-soluble and works best when taken with oily or fatty foods. Look for a soft gel, liquid, or oil form with a small amount of vitamin E added.

Colostrum stimulates the immune system and is an effective all-natural antibiotic. It is available in health food stores as a capsule or lozenge. It's best absorbed if taken as a lozenge (Shomali and Wolfsthal 1997).

Ginkgo biloba is an extract made from the leaves of the ginkgo tree. It apparently improves general blood circulation and thus may be of some help in treating Alzheimer's disease symptoms. Studies are underway to learn whether it can delay or prevent dementia in older people (Kleijnen and Knipschild 1992). There is no evidence that ginkgo will cure or prevent Alzheimer's.

Caution: Ginkgo biloba is also an anticoagulant and should be used with caution if taken with a daily dose of 81 or more mg aspirin, which has the same blood-thinning effect (Sierpina, Wollschlaeger, and Blumenthal 2003).

Glucosamine chondroitin sometimes works wonders restoring joint cartilage damaged by arthritis.

Gotu kola is good for heart and liver health as well as for cardiovascular and circulatory functions. It also stimulates the nervous system and improves poor appetite and mental function.

Lecithin is a very important source of choline and inositol, two important antioxidants in the B-vitamin family. Both choline and inositol are classified as B vitamins. Lecithin is also crucial to the breakdown of cholesterol.

Lutein is a yellow pigment found in our eyes. It acts as a light filter and an antioxidant that protects optic nerves and has numerous other health benefits. The best natural source for lutein is spinach and other dark green leafy vegetables.

Rosemary helps circulatory problems and irregular blood pressure. It also has anticancer and antitumor properties.

St. John's wort can help nerve pain and depression. It is a good alternative to prescription antidepressants. However, do not use without consulting your physician. This herb sometimes has adverse effects in people who suffer from serious arthritis or an immune-system deficiency.

(*See also:* Alzheimer's Medications; Dementia; Diet and Nutrition; Eye and Sight Health; Health; Vitamins)

■ ■ ■ ■ ■ ■ ■
Alzheimer's Disease

Alzheimer's disease is named after Dr. Alois Alzheimer, the German neuropathologist who identified the disease in 1906. A patient of his at a local mental institution had exhibited severe dementia for ten years before dying at the age of fifty-five. When an autopsy was performed on her brain, Dr. Alzheimer found tangled nerve cells and plaque deposits that he believed to be the cause of her dementia. *Alzheimer's disease* is the term for a specific kind of deterioration of nerve clusters in the brain. These clusters become calcified and tangled, causing many brain cells to die.

There are between four and a half and six million victims of Alzheimer's disease in this country. With the aging of our population, these numbers are expected to increase dramatically. According to the Alzheimer's Association, about 10 percent of everyone over sixty-five and about half of everyone over the age of eighty-five has Alzheimer's.

A person will live an average of eight years following diagnosis. In the past twenty years, research has been stepped up dramatically, but we continue to have many more questions than answers. Some medications on the market can ease or delay symptoms for some folks. There are some promising developments in the search for a vaccine, but it will probably be years before these are ready to use on people.

CAUSES   Researchers have identified multiple factors associated with Alzheimer's disease, among them genetic connections, biochemical changes, and environmental factors, such as head trauma in the patient's past, alcohol abuse, and toxins. However the basic cause, if there is just one, remains elusive.

> *The heart and stroke connection.* Studies show that people with heart disease, high blood pressure, a history of strokes and elevated cholesterol are at considerably greater risk for developing Alzheimer's disease (Sparks et al. 2000). Ministrokes, also known as TIAs (transient ischaemic attacks), damage the blood vessels in the brain and often

lead to multi-infarct dementia, which mimics and may eventually lead to Alzheimer's disease.

The genetic connection. Gene mutations of three chromosomes (1, 14, and 21) have been identified as being responsible for early onset Alzheimer's, which strikes people in their thirties to fifties. However, together these three chromosomes account for only a small percentage of all Alzheimer's cases (about 5 percent). A fourth gene, *APOE*, found on chromosome 19, shows up in 65 percent of all Alzheimer's patients studied (Tanzi and Parson 2000). This particular gene helps to transport cholesterol in the bloodstream. It comes in different forms. One form appears to prevent the development of Alzheimer's, while another, *APOE4*, seems to create more susceptibility to the disease. Note, however, that many people with *APOE4* don't develop the disease. At this point in time, there are no explanations for why some people develop the disease and others don't. Even if your parent has Alzheimer's disease linked to genetic causes, there's no guarantee that you'll get it.

The protein connection. Amyloid beta protein occurs naturally in large quantities in the brain. It enters the cell plasma and decomposes. When this protein doesn't break down properly, it accumulates, destroys the cells, and causes neurological damage (Sunderland et al. 2003). The greater the degree of dementia, the higher the levels of these proteins. Another protein, tau, is also found in the nerve tangles typical in Alzheimer's. These are important discoveries in the search for more accurate tests, vaccines, and antidotes for the disease once it has begun to develop (Huang et al. 2000). Numerous studies show an unusually high accumulation of amyloid beta protein in Alzheimer's brains as well as the protein named tau.

The folate and choline deficiency connection. There is a correlation between a deficiency in folic acid (folate is one of the B vitamins) and Alzheimer's disease. Vitamin B_{12} deficiency can also cause a distinct type of dementia (Cummings and Cole 2002). Unfortunately, this condition is not reversible once the disease has developed. Folate is found in legumes, salmon, tuna, citrus fruit, and root vegetables. (Cooking destroys it.) Vitamin B_{12} is found only in animal foods such as milk, eggs, and most meat, especially liver.

Another B vitamin, choline, is crucial to the health of nerve transmitters in the brain and other organs. Some research is showing that serious choline deficiency is common in Alzheimer's victims. Choline deficiency impairs the nervous system and brain function as well as the digestive system and blood pressure. Choline is found in meat, egg yolks, legumes, soybeans, and whole grain cereals (Kaplan 1992).

The aluminum connection. Aluminum is one of the most abundant minerals on earth and we consume an average of 30 to 50 mg a day through our intake of foods and water. Upon autopsy, four times the normal amount of aluminum deposit is found in Alzheimer's brains. There's disagreement among scientists and researchers as to the significance of this fact. You may want to take precautions anyway and avoid excessive exposure to the metal. That can be done easily if you have your drinking water tested and avoid storing and cooking acidic foods in aluminum containers (Werbach 1993).

Environmental toxins. There appears to be some correlation between the use of herbicides (weed killers) and insecticides (bug sprays) and the development of Alzheimer's. Anecdotal evidence points to Alzheimer's being more prevalent among persons who have been exposed excessively to household cleaners. Environment and lifestyle may play an equal or greater role than genetics in the development of Alzheimer's. These factors include nutrition, head injuries, and exposure to pollutants ranging from herbicides, insecticides, and air pollution to household chemicals and cosmetics. These contaminants elevate free radicals in our systems, causing oxidation,

which in turn interferes with healthy cell development
(Blaylock 2002).

TESTS   Someone showing symptoms of dementia should undergo a
thorough physical, including basic blood tests to detect possible
deficient levels of folate, B_{12}, and thyroid hormones. Once it has been
ascertained that the dementia is not caused by a reversible condition,
the next step is testing by a neurologist or psychologist, who will use
verbal memory tests and most likely order an MRI or a CAT scan.
Researchers are currently working on simple skin and urine tests.
These tests should soon be available to the general medical
community (Royce 2002; Pratico 2001).

VACCINES   There is cautious optimism about the progress of finding
an Alzheimer's vaccine. The drugs under investigation are thought to
stimulate the immune system to "recognize" and attack the amyloid
plaques that are identified with Alzheimer's brain abnormalities
(Hock et al. 2002). Human tests have been promising, although the
initial rounds were halted due to side effects in several subjects.
Subsequent tests did show that the vaccine had, in fact, been
successful in slowing the progression of the disease. It will take
several more human trials to learn if these substances are safe and
effective as vaccines.

There is also cautious optimism about another Alzheimer's vaccine currently under development. Researchers have identified a substance that successfully prevents the formation of plaques in aged
laboratory animals. It even shows signs of dissolving existing plaques.
Human tests are under way. So far, there have been no serious side
effects in human subjects. It will take several years to learn if these
substances are effective as vaccines. The Alzheimer's community
expresses caution, reminding us that many good results with animal
subjects from other promising vaccines (such as those for diabetes)
have not been effective with human beings.

(*See also:* Alternative Remedies; Dementia; Diet and
Nutrition; Health; Vitamins)

Alzheimer's Disease

■ ■ ■ ■ ■ ■ ■ ■

A

Alzheimer's Medications

There are several Alzheimer's medications available. Although we're still not able to cure or reverse the disease, these medications help many Alzheimer's people with their general well-being. Problems like agitation, sleeplessness, and depression are minimized.

The most frequently prescribed medications are Aricept (donepezil), Exelon (rivastigmine tartrate), Cognex (tacrine), and Reminyl (galantamine hydrobromide), which all act to increase acetylcholine levels in the brain. Loss of acetylcholine-producing neurons is linked to Alzheimer's, but it's still not clear why these medicines work.

Aricept, Exelon, and Reminyl essentially all provide the same benefits of delaying cognition decline and improving an Alzheimer's person's quality of life. Gastric problems are, however, possible side effects for all three medications. Consult your doctor to find out which one might work best for your particular Alzheimer's person.

Most physicians recommend that Alzheimer's patients start on one of these medications when they're first diagnosed and remain on it for the duration, if they're tolerated, although some insurance companies will stop paying for these medications when the disease is considered severe. The Alzheimer's Association sometimes offers grants in such cases. (See Resources for Web site and phone number.)

Note: Some studies show that the benefits of Aricept are greatly increased when taken with vitamin E. According to a study concluded in 2003 by Alzheimer's researcher Dr. David Beversdorf of Ohio State University, the benefits of Aricept are greatly increased when taken along with vitamin E (Klatte et al. 2003).

Cognex (tacrine). This was the first Alzheimer's medication on the market, but it is no longer being marketed aggressively because of the risk of liver damage. Monthly blood tests are usually necessary for anyone on this medication.

Memantine. The newest addition to the Alzheimer's pharmacy is memantine, sold under the brand names of Namenda and Ebixa. Memantine provides benefits to those in the middle and late stages of the disease. It helps to maintain the ability to communicate and independently dress and bathe for longer periods of time. Because this drug addresses a different brain function, it can be taken along with Aricept, Exelon, or Reminyl for an even greater benefit.

Estrogen. Hormone replacement therapies (HRT) were previously thought to help prevent or slow the onset of Alzheimer's disease. The Women's Health Initiative Memory Study (WHIMS) on memory actually showed cognitive decline with estrogen plus progesterone. (Shaywitz and Shaywitz 2000). So far, there's no clear evidence that estrogen alone is beneficial, and recent studies have shown many other negative effects from these drugs (Sarrel 2002). Doctors no longer want to prescribe them for the purpose of preventing Alzheimer's or any other form of cognitive decline.

NSAIDs (nonsteroidal anti-inflammatory drugs). A history of using NSAIDs, such as ibuprofen, has been correlated with a decreased risk of Alzheimer's disease, but the reason for this is not known (Aisen et al. 2003). The thinking is that NSAIDs help to reduce inflammation in an Alzheimer's person's brain and thus slows the progression of the disease. Studies are currently underway to see if NSAIDs do, in fact, slow the progression of the disease.

Caution: Ulcers and bleeding in the stomach may appear in 15 to 20 percent of those who take daily doses of NSAIDs for chronic illnesses. These medications can also cause kidney problems, especially in the elderly. There are also concerns about the interactions of NSAIDs with other medications.

Vitamin E. Research has shown that vitamin E slows the progress of some of the consequences of Alzheimer's disease (Zandi et al. 2004). Scientists now are studying vitamin E to learn whether it can prevent or delay the disease in patients with mild cognitive impairment. Be sure to check with your doctor before using any over-the-counter products.

(*See also:* Alternative Remedies; Dementia; Diet and Nutrition; Health; Vitamins)

■ ■ ■ ■ ■ ■ ■ ■

Appetite

Dad's appetite has changed. Sometimes he'll barely touch his lunch, while at other times it seems he won't stop eating. His dementia actually may affect his feelings of hunger and satiation, so he has no sense of when and how much to eat. If you are in this situation, here are some questions to ask yourself:

› Is his medication affecting his appetite?

› Is he having elimination problems?

› Is he having dental problems?

› Is he suffering from aches and pains?

› Is he getting a proper amount of good exercise?

› Is his spirit otherwise good?

› Is he showing signs of depression?

› Is he forgetting how to use eating utensils?

If none of these is a problem, these food issues are probably due to his Alzheimer's. You can help him by changing your approach to your cooking and mealtimes. If your dad is ravenous one day, then cook him an enormous breakfast, and if he's only interested in snacks the next day, why not let him snack? Why do we have to eat three square meals every day, anyway?

In the meantime, you can monitor his overall food consumption to ensure that he's getting his basic dietary requirements. Make sure he gets his daily vitamins and, when necessary, use supplements. Be aware that popular supplement drinks are often very high in sugar. If this problem persists and you're concerned about it, talk to his doctor.

(*See also:* Depression; Diet and Nutrition; Eating; Exercise; Health)

■ ■ ■ ■ ■ ■ ■ ■

Attitude

As you read through this book, you'll find that the central theme is maintaining a positive attitude. It's not always easy, but by taking a lighthearted approach to your daily situations, you'll discover that your grandmother often responds more favorably. She reflects your moods and actions. It's also important for you to be aware of how her memory and thinking have changed. Often she's living in an altered reality, having regressed back to the comfortable memories of her childhood. When you adapt your reactions to her reality, you'll find her much more cooperative.

Alzheimer's disease has changed your grandmother's personality. She often does or says things that would have been totally out of character before she developed the disease. She cannot control her moods or feelings and, more than ever, she needs your support and acceptance. Sometimes you may find it difficult to control your own reactions, but you are constantly reminded that Grandma mirrors your moods by her behavior.

There are times when you want to fly off the handle, but you control yourself with deep breathing. And, if things get really bad and you think you may explode, go to another room or outside for a break. No matter what happens, try to remember that this is Alzheimer's disease and your grandmother is no longer in control of her behavior. However, you can influence her with your attitude.

Decide what is really most important at the moment. Often, you may have to set aside your old ideas of what is proper and concentrate on Grandma's needs from her perspective. If she is very agitated, your unruffled demeanor will help to calm her down. You may have to fake your initial reaction, because it can be very hard to accept that your grandmother can behave like this. After she has settled down again, use one of your effective diversions to get her into a positive state of mind.

You will find yourself changing your ideas about what's important and your focus will turn to the enjoyment of sharing small everyday pleasures with Grandma. And don't forget that humor and a lighthearted attitude will get you over many hurdles. Limit your humorous comments to things that she finds funny. There will be times when she either does or says something sweetly funny. Hard as it may be at the moment, make sure you never laugh at her.

Begin each day with an upbeat greeting: "Good morning to you, good morning to you . . . (to the tune of Happy Birthday). We're going to have a special day today! Let's start with a good breakfast. Breakfast is the most important meal of the day! That's what my grandmother always said. . . . Oh, that's right, you are my grandmother!"

Use encouraging remarks throughout the day to reinforce these good feelings. Remarks like the following can be very encouraging:

"I'm so glad you thought of this."

"I'm so happy we can share this. It's so much better when we do this together."

"Aren't we lucky that we have each other?"

You'll also want to take care of yourself. Take time out with respite care assistance and the support of your family and friends.

And, above all other concerns, try to maintain your sense of humor, because sometimes it will be the only thing that will keep you from going completely crazy.

You're often frustrated by others' attitudes, so you have to become an advocate for Grandma. In public places you've learned to ignore the occasional insensitive stare. When it comes to dealing with the outside world, you're becoming her spokesperson and you stand up on her behalf when she's confronted with patronizing or demeaning remarks or behavior from strangers.

(*See also:* Acceptance; Baby Talk; Conversations; Dignity; Diversions; Empathy; Normal; Questions; Reactions; Validation)

B

■ ■ ■ ■ ■ ■ ■ ■

Baby Talk

There are some people who resort to baby talk anytime they encounter someone whom they perceive as weak or ill. They don't realize how degrading it is to the person with whom they're speaking, let alone how idiotic they make themselves sound when they talk that way. To speak in this manner to anyone except a baby, or perhaps a lover, is insulting, demeaning, and just plain rude. The most difficult situations often arise because some of the most well-meaning people don't realize that their tone of voice is patronizing.

If someone starts baby talking or cooing with your mom, you can deal with it effectively by saying, "I'm sorry, but my mother relates best when you talk to her in a normal adult voice."

Let's suppose that you and your mother are out for an afternoon stroll, and you bump into an old acquaintance of yours. She's an effusive personality who bubbles uncontrollably. She beams at you like a spotlight, while she gushes, "Oh, are you and your mother out for a little walk?" in a little girl's voice. Then, she turns to Mom and pats her arm patronizingly as she gushes some more nonsense to you. "Isn't that sweet of you to take your Mommy out for walkies!" Finally, she addresses your mother directly and says, "Don't you look cute today, dearie. What a sweet dress, it's just precious on you."

The look on your mother's face says it all: she is confused and upset. You'll have to do something. You could give this woman a taste of her own rude medicine and say, "Well, Dahling, what brings you out into this revealing daylight? I must say that old dress still looks good on you!"

However, you might be uncomfortable using this kind of snide language, and this woman is probably too self-absorbed to get your message anyway. Instead, tell her in plain English: "My mother is a mature adult. She does not appreciate it when people use baby talk to talk to her."

(*See also:* Attitude; Comprehension; Conversations; Dignity; Normal)

■ ■ ■ ■ ■ ■ ■ ■
Bathroom

It's important for your sister to continue using the toilet by herself for as long as possible. If it's necessary for you to supervise, remain calm and straightforward as you coach her through the motions. For example, before going out, you could say something like this: "Let's use the toilet now, before we go out. You go first; and I'll go after you. We can share a flush and save two and a half gallons of water that way!"

If she hesitates or seems confused about her clothes or the toilet itself, you can gently direct her in this manner: Point to the toilet and say, "Here's the toilet. Pull down your pants and underwear. Pull them down to your knees. There. Now you can sit down on the toilet. Let me give you a hand."

She may need guidance or physical assistance, so you want to be careful in the way you word your comments, so she can't answer, "No." For example, if you say, "Here's the toilet, would you like me to help you?" she's likely to say, "No."

Instead, use language that doesn't call for any answer: "Here's the toilet. I'll give you a hand."

If you can, sit on the tub or a chair next to her and chat. Then ask her if she has finished peeing or if she needs to take a "BM," or whatever term is familiar to her. Hand her the toilet tissue when she's finished and talk her through her motions:

"Here's some tissue to wipe with. Go ahead and wipe yourself down there." You may need to demonstrate on yourself: "See, this is how you do it. There, you're all finished! Great! After you pull up your underwear and pants, it's my turn to pee."

Have her stay in the bathroom with you or keep the door open while you pee, so she'll be reassured to see that you go through the same motions. Using the toilet is a perfectly natural function. You'll build trust and confidence by sharing the experience with her whenever you can.

One morning as you're helping your sister to dress, you might notice that her nails are coated with a brown substance. It may suddenly dawn on you that she has been scratching her anus. Maybe she can't figure out how to use the toilet paper anymore, or maybe she's constipated and has been trying to free herself of her stool. This is not unusual behavior for Alzheimer's people. In fact, it's common. In the future, make it a point to check her hands discreetly after she's used the toilet. You can use moist wipes to wipe her bottom and hands before you help her finish washing up. You might say, "Let's see, Sweetheart, we'd better wash this brown stuff off your hands. I'll run some water for you and you can let your hands soak for a minute. Might as well let the water do the work, right? Now you want to use some of this soap. There, you're as good as new!"

If this problem persists, talk to her doctor about putting her on a regimen of stool softener, fiber supplement, and increased liquid intake. You might also have her checked for hemorrhoids, which can make elimination troublesome.

> **Tip!** If your sister has trouble finding or using the toilet paper holder, get a standing paper towel holder, set it on the counter or on the floor next to the toilet, and use it for toilet tissue. It's bigger and easier to see. Also, she may not be familiar with liquid soap, so keep a regular bar of soap at the sink.

(See also: Coaching; Compliments; Home Safety; Questions)

■ ■ ■ ■ ■ ■ ■ ■
Bath Time

As Grandma grows more dependent on you and others, she will feel her self-determination slipping away. There will be a few activities left that will allow her some semblance of control: bathing, eating, and dressing. Suppose you've become quite adept at helping Grandma with bathing, shampooing, and drying off. Everything seems to be going so well, but suddenly one afternoon at bath time, she lashes out at you, losing her temper and calling you names. What's the best way to handle this situation?

Before you decide to tackle giving her a bath, ask yourself these questions:

> ‣ Does she really need a bath today?

> ‣ How frequently did she bathe in the past?

Most Americans bathe or shower daily, but Grandma's from a generation that bathed only when necessary. You may recall her telling you years ago how her family took their weekly baths. These days she's often living in the altered reality of her childhood, so you might want to consider giving her a bath once or twice a week instead of every day. You can use details from her stories about her childhood to help her feel more secure about bathing. For example, you might say something like, "When I was a little kid, you used to tell me about how you had to take a bath in a big tin tub, and your mother would heat the water on top of the stove because you didn't have hot running water. You got to take a bath only once a week, because it was so much work. Nowadays we have hot water coming out of the tap. We're lucky, aren't we?"

She also may have very strong feelings about the time of day that she takes her bath. For instance, if she usually bathed on Saturday mornings, then you can choose to bathe her in the morning, and that will feel okay to her.

She may not remember what the bathing or showering procedure is. So, when you ask her if she wants to take a bath, her first impulse may be to refuse firmly so she won't have to tackle all those strange procedures that seem scary and uncertain to her. If she says no to taking a bath, you can decide to change your approach.

Instead of asking her, try this alternative scenario:

"Grandma, let me help you up."

"Why?"

"Come, I'll show you."

If she resists, talk about something unrelated while you help her out of her chair. Continue talking to her as you casually lead her to the bathroom. When you get there, you might say something like this: "Yesterday, when we went to the store, you found a wonderful new shampoo. You told me you wanted to try it today, so I'm going to turn on the shower for you so you can use it on your hair. I'll be glad to help you with your shower."

She might respond, "I don't need a shower! I'm not dirty!" But you could answer that by saying, "Oh, I know you're not dirty, but today's Saturday and that's your favorite shower day. Here we are! Here, smell this great shampoo. Your hair will smell so good, won't it?"

Coach her step-by-step into the shower and help her seat herself on the shower stool. After she's seated, turn on the water and let her feel it streaming over her body from the hand-held shower. Keep adjusting it until she's pleased with the temperature. Patiently and cheerfully coach her through the process. You'll want to encourage her to do as much as she can by herself. After she's dressed, tell her again how good she looks and how sweet her hair smells. Then celebrate the successful bath by suggesting something like, "Let's have a cup of tea and a chocolate chip cookie. How does that sound?"

As you relax with her, share an intimate conversation. By creating a relaxed environment, you will establish bath time as a positive experience. If you stick to a routine that includes these comfortable connections, you'll build up trust and minimize problems down the road.

Keep a variety of soaps, shampoos, and towels on hand, and take shopping excursions to buy new shampoo or soap. If you encourage her to make the selection, later you can honestly admire her excellent choice.

(*See also:* Coaching; Compliments; Home Safety; Questions)

■ ■ ■ ■ ■ ■ ■ ■

Birthdays

Your friend Tom probably doesn't remember his chronological age, because nobody "feels" a certain age. Think about it. We feel tired. We feel energetic. We feel ill. But we don't "feel" a particular age. If anything, we relate age to well-being out of habit. We say things like,

"I feel a hundred years old, I am so tired!" or "I feel great today, positively like a teenager!"

Let's suppose you're hosting a party for Tom's birthday, complete with balloons, ice cream, and cake with lots of candles. Many of your friends have come to help celebrate. One of the guests cheerfully, but insensitively, exclaims to Tom, "Wow, you are ninety-one today! How does that feel?" Tom may respond to that by looking stricken and confused. Ninety-one is very old! Even a person with dementia knows that. If that's Tom's response, you can quickly go to his side, put your arms around him, and cheerfully say, "Tom, we are having a birthday party for you today. Which birthday would you like to celebrate?"

He might respond enthusiastically with "twenty-eight!"

That's the birthday you'll be celebrating.

(*See also:* Age; Humor)

■ ■ ■ ■ ■ ■ ■ ■
Body Language

Grandpa may have a hard time expressing himself. You're becoming accustomed to observing his more subtle gestures and expressions and learning to anticipate his needs and feelings. As you become increasingly attuned to his nonverbal communication, a private language may develop between the two of you. The unexpected bonus of caring for a person with Alzheimer's is that, often, you learn to feel closer to that person while learning to interpret the subtle signs of nonverbal communication.

Sometimes your grandmother may look slightly anxious and distracted as she pats the sides of her pants, where normally there would be a pocket. But you reach for a tissue and hand it to her and she blows her nose while smiling gratefully. She may have trouble remembering words for common items, but fortunately you've become familiar with much of her body language. She tends to make a certain little squirming motion when she needs the toilet, and twists her mouth in

B

a particular way when she's thirsty. And when it's nap time, she gets this far-away look in her eyes that says she's sleepy.

Suppose you're both in the car and Grandma's too fidgety to settle down. She has a vacant look in her eyes, so you say, "You look as if you're hot. Would you like me to open the window?"

She might respond by mumbling and nodding. So, as you go through the motions, describe to her what you are doing to reassure her. You could say, "See. I push a button over here and your window rolls down. Magic, huh? That's better, isn't it? The fresh air sure smells good, doesn't it? You'll let me know if it's too windy for you, won't you?"

You know that chances are pretty slim that she'll be able to let you know. She may not be able to express it, but every time you notice how she's feeling and address her situation, you give her a feeling of control. You learn to watch her out of the corner of your eye to make sure she's doing all right.

(*See also*: Empathy; Health; Hearing Health;
Incontinence; Pain; Walking)

C

■ ■ ■ ■ ■ ■ ■ ■
Care Facilities

Most of us pay little attention to long-term care facilities until the need arises. Even if you never have to face the possibility with family members, it's a good idea to familiarize yourself now with the choices available in your community. The best Alzheimer's homes offer the comforts and atmosphere of a private home. Memory-impaired persons are not sick as such, and they don't need a hospital-like setting. As you tour a facility, ask yourself this question: Would I want to live here?

CATEGORIES   Every state in the union has offices or departments that deal especially with issues of the elderly: Look for your State Agency on Aging, Adult Protective Services, and licensing agencies. Give any one of them a call, ask questions, get opinions, and learn your state's requirements for different types of facilities.

> *Independent living.* Usually apartment-type complexes. Minimal personal care. Unlicensed and unregulated. Some meals and light housekeeping are usually included in monthly fees.

> *Assisted living.* Some personal care, usually state licensed. Meals, personal hygiene, housekeeping, and some laundry should be included in the monthly fees. Most assisted-living facilities have resident nurses to supervise and dispense medication. Many assisted living facilities offer an Alzheimer's wing.

C

Nursing homes. Full nursing care, federally regulated, and state licensed. Medicaid eligible.

Alzheimer's homes. Full care for special-needs residents, state licensed. Note that in some states, homes for Alzheimer's patients are Medicaid eligible.

When you examine a facility, be sure to check out the following aspects and services.

Activities   Request copies of the activities schedule. Indoor and outdoor activities should include a variety of exercise programs and group events centered on music, art, and intellectual stimulation. The activity programs should reflect the various levels, interests, and abilities of the residents, with opportunities for individual creative expression. Residents should be encouraged to engage in projects beyond the scheduled programs: for example, setting tables, assisting with cooking, folding laundry, sorting books, watering flowers, feeding resident animals, and so forth.

Evaluation   If the day comes when you must move a family member into a facility, ask to see its criteria for placing residents and assess the qualifications of those making the determination. Many facilities will gladly give you an "evaluation," but be aware that some may be more interested in filling a bed than in giving you an accurate assessment. Get a second opinion, either from your local advocate for the aged or from a trusted physician with a specialty in geriatrics.

Nutrition   Request a copy of the menu for a week. Menus should reflect a nutritious, well-rounded diet including plenty of vegetables and fruit, which are also available or served as snacks throughout the day along with juices and water. The residents should have plenty of time to eat their meals without being rushed and receive help from staff when needed, such as guidance with eating utensils.

It's perfectly acceptable for you to request to eat lunch with the residents. This will give you the opportunity to observe typical interactions between staff and residents.

Care Facilities

Physical Facilities   Whether large or small, the best Alzheimer's facilities are "user-friendly" homes. You want the place to be attractive, but ask yourself this question: Is the place designed for the residents or is it designed to impress visitors like yourself? The furniture, color schemes, and decorations should appear to be chosen for the pleasure and comfort of the residents. The furniture should be selected for the comfort of the elderly, easy to get in and out of. Furniture, including wheelchairs, should be grouped to encourage conversations and socializing. The residents should have free and safe access to all the major living areas, indoors and out. Music and television should be chosen for the pleasure of the residents. The comfort level of room temperature is important, it should be at least 75 degrees Fahrenheit. As we age, our body temperature drops an average of one degree and generally we don't move a lot. That's why elderly folks are often cold.

Hopefully there will be signs of creativity and fun: books, games, flowers (albeit silk flowers), and residents' artworks displayed with respect and pride. Progressive facilities also have pets and gardens for residents to tend.

Individual apartments or rooms should be attractively decorated and personalized as much as space will allow. Shared or semiprivate rooms can still offer privacy and personal touches, such as family photographs on the walls. Note that many Alzheimer's patients receive a lot of benefit from shared rooms, because of the security of having a friend in the other bed.

Residents   The chief priority for any facility should be the residents' quality of life. Many Alzheimer's and nursing homes today are adopting person-centered care, where the emphasis is on the immediate emotional needs of their residents. This sometimes means forgoing making the beds to help a resident cope with a crisis situation, or serving several small meals over the course of one day instead of the usual three squares.

The residents' quality of life can be hard to detect on a brief visit. Ask the aides if they're encouraged to adapt themselves to the residents' needs. The residents should be dressed in clean, comfortable clothing appropriate to the time of day and they should appear to be comfortable and content and interact to the best of their ability.

C

You should witness frequent and positive interactions between staff and the residents. For example, if a staff member encounters a resident in the process of doing her work, she should acknowledge this person, even if it's only a simple "Hi!"

Staff Staff members should be at ease when you talk to them. Hopefully, you'll observe members of the staff interacting with residents. They should be using normal conversational tones, without condescending baby talk. They should handle agitated residents with calm, gentle diversions, and without reprimands.

Find out the number of staff who work directly with residents. Six residents for each staff member is a decent ratio. Also, ask about special qualifications of the staff, such as CNA (certified nurse's assistant) certification. Request a schedule of classes for the staff and list of topics, especially for Alzheimer's disease and communication skills. Appropriate training sessions should be mandatory for the entire staff, including housekeeping and maintenance staff. These classes should be *in-service*, meaning they're given during the work-day or that staff members are paid to attend the classes after hours.

Inquire about the number of contract or part-time employees. Contract employees and part-time employees usually have no bene-fits such as sick days, paid vacations, and health care or medical cov-erage. The presence or absence of such benefits is a good indication of a facility's level of commitment to its staff. And the following rela-tionships usually hold true:

As management does to staff, staff does to residents.

A FINAL WORD When you have tentatively chosen a place, request time to observe the facility's operations on your own. Spend enough time there for the staff to get used to your presence so that they will go about their normal business without paying too much attention to you. Sit in on activity sessions and eat a meal or two with the residents. Observe the staff. Spend time with the residents. That way you are more likely to find out what your family member's new living arrangement will really be like.

Good luck! And remember that, even if you find the perfect facility, it's imperative that you still remain the center of your family member's life. Visit often, share meals with him or her, participate in conversations with his or her friends there, and take your family member on outings as much as is possible.

(*See also*: Environment; Transitions)

■ ■ ■ ■ ■ ■ ■ ■

Celebrations

Human beings thrive on rituals. All cultures celebrate major holidays, whether it is Feast Day, Chanukah, Kwanzaa, Ramadan, New Year's Eve, or Christmas. To a greater or lesser degree there are always cookies, decorations, candles, feasting, and presents. All at once! No wonder celebrations seem like a magic time.

Your mother always took great pride in her special Christmas cookies. The recipe has been handed down for generations and includes a secret ingredient. Now she's no longer sure what kind of cookies they were, but she will still describe the process in minute detail.

Suppose that on a hot summer's day, Mom declares that she must start baking her traditional Christmas cookies immediately. Don't discourage her. Who says you can't celebrate Christmas in July or April? Put up the lights, bake cookies, light candles, and wrap presents with colorful ribbons. Other family members may need some persuading to sing Christmas carols on a sweltering summer day, but once you've adjusted yourselves to this topsy-turvy world, you're all guaranteed to have a good time.

You can create new rituals and celebrations anytime you want (or need) one. You can have a "Friendship Party" to celebrate your living together or a "First Day of Spring Party." A "We Cleaned out the Dresser Party" can follow a "Second Day of Spring Party." At other times, you can create small daily celebrations by dressing up the kitchen with a special tablecloth, a bouquet of flowers, and a plate of goodies. You may want to add a surprise gift now and then. You can keep a stash of gift-wrapped boxes in a closet for just such occasions. The boxes can be recycled back into the closet.

(*See also*: Birthdays; Humor; Laughter; Validation)

■ ■ ■ ■ ■ ■ ■ ■
Children

Children are often able to communicate without hang-ups or prejudices. They can get past illogical conversations and move into a realm of feelings and deeper understanding. Some nursing homes have their staff's children visit for a day, while others arrange visits from schools on a regular basis. A few advanced homes combine their facilities with full-time children's day-care centers. The resulting interactions have been very beneficial for the elderly and children alike.

Ellen's grandchildren live out of town and can see her only a couple of times a year, hardly enough visits for someone who's always loved being around kids. So, you've occasionally borrowed your friends' grandchildren to come along when you visit her. Then one day, while on one of your walks around the neighborhood, Ellen struck up a conversation with a five-year-old who lives a few houses down the street.

Since then the two of them have developed a special relationship. They spend time together in the garden, counting the petals on flowers and arguing over images they see in the clouds. Ellen chats away, telling stories that don't make much sense to you, but her five-year-old companion is totally engrossed. The little one brings her toys and books that the two of them read together. You serve them cookies and ice cream and appreciate having a respite.

The visits have an uplifting and invigorating effect on Ellen, and her five-year-old friend is delighted with an adult's undivided attention. She seems oblivious to Ellen's communication problems and accepts her, confusion, garbled speech, and all. When her young pal can't visit, you and Ellen go on picnics at the neighborhood playground to watch the children play. On cloudy days, you visit the children's department of the local library together and listen to the librarian read fairy tales to the kids. You even take Ellen to a fast-food restaurant where she focuses on a toddler and asks the mother, in the sweetest tone of voice, "Would you by any chance allow us to cuddle that beautiful baby of yours?"

When you and Ellen leave the restaurant, the baby is cooing and the proud mother is beaming with delight.

(*See also:* Attitude; Empathy; Games; Singing)

Choices

Someone with dementia typically has problems holding several thoughts at one time, so when you offer choices, try to limit yourself to two clear choices at a time. You may have to repeat or rephrase them to help the person grasp what is meant.

For example, your wife's always been an independent and opinionated woman. Now that you have to make decisions for her in most areas of her life, try to provide her with as much self-determination as possible by giving her choices as often as you can. When she's getting dressed, you can hold up two shirts and let her pick the one she wants to wear. You could ask, "Let's see . . . you have this blue-checked shirt and this pink flowered one. Which one would you like to wear today?"

At breakfast you can offer her a choice of how she wants her eggs cooked, and you try to describe the choice in specific terms since she may not remember them herself: "I can fix your eggs sunny-side up or scrambled. Would you like them scrambled?"

If your wife has great difficulty expressing herself, you can rephrase the choices you're offering so she can respond with a simple yes or no. For example, if you say to her, "I promised you that we would go for a drive today. We can go to the library or we can go to your favorite art gallery. How about the library?" and she responds with "No," you could say, "Well, it sounds like you'd rather go to the gallery today. Is that right?" Then she might answer, "Yes."

(*See also:* Coaching; Communication; Questions)

Coaching

Grandma's confusion often makes it difficult for her to perform even simple tasks. Her brain no longer processes incoming information in the same way yours does. You can help her out by coaching her, verbally and physically. As you talk her through a process, be extra conscious to keep your tone on an adult level, which is more difficult in

C

these situations because it can be heartbreaking to watch a loved one be so helpless.

Any movements our bodies make involve subconscious planning. We dash down a busy sidewalk at rush hour and we don't stumble over the curb or bump into other people. As we go through the process of walking, our subconscious minds are constantly surveying and memorizing the terrain ahead. Grandma is no longer able to process these subconscious impressions. She walks with hesitation and uncertainty because of her inability to plan ahead. You have become her "movement guide" as you describe out loud what's a few steps ahead, leading her gently by the arm.

Suppose you are going to take a drive and Grandma looks at you in bewilderment. She has no idea of how to get into the car. She needs your help, so you take her through the motions with gentle coaching. Approach this as though it's the first time she's ever gotten into a car. Guide her step-by-step in a clear voice. Use gestures and demonstrate how it is done as much as is possible. Say, "This is your seat" (as you pat the seat). "First you step in here with this foot" (as you pat her left leg), "then you sit down on the seat. I'll support you so you won't fall. Now pull your other foot in and move over to the middle of the seat. Perfect! There, you did it!"

The next time you go for a drive, you'll probably have to go through the whole process all over again. With practice, your coaching will become as smooth as a flight attendant's safety spiel. Always make sure that you are clear and precise, without sounding patronizing.

You're getting used to talking your way through most of the things you do with or around Grandma. At first, it was awkward and it made you feel kind of silly to think out loud, but now this new skill helps you to coach her when necessary:

"Let me see, I'm going to change the linen before we go for a drive, okay? Would you like to give me a hand? . . . Here's your clean sheet. Would you hold that while I remove the dirty one . . . There, now may I have the clean one please? . . . I'm going to slip this far corner on the mattress first, then this one . . . now I'll pull it and fit it over the foot of your bed . . . what do you think? Does it look good to you?"

Ask for Grandma's opinion often, even if she's not coherent or her answer has no relation to your question. Simply respond as if she's offered an excellent idea, but don't go overboard in your positive reaction. Try to keep it low-key and sincere.

———————————

C

You've coached your friend Molly through all sorts of everyday tasks, from how to use the toilet to how to button her blouse. You've discovered that your coaching goes easier if you alter your vocabulary and your guidance methods. Molly's often confused about left and right, so you've learned to rephrase directions by saying "this one" and "the other." For example, to help Molly dress, you say, "Are you ready to put on your shirt? Here, put one arm into this sleeve" (as you hold it open for her), "and then your other arm into the other sleeve." And "Here are your shoes. Put this foot into the first one" (as you pat the correct foot) ". . . and your other foot into this other one."

When Molly sees a spoon, she may not remember what it is, so she's not able to prepare her hand to grab it. You can help her by placing the spoon in her hand until she or her fingers remember what to do. You say, "Here's your soup. This is the soupspoon. You can hold it in this hand" (as you place the spoon in her hand).

Molly may have forgotten the words for the parts of her body, so whenever you need her to do something specific, you can help her connect by patting her on her limb as you use the correct term. For example, say, "I'm going to turn on the water for your shower. Feel it with your hand" (as you pat her hand), "and let me know if it feels comfortable to you."

Other directions may baffle her, such as "turn around" or "face" in a certain direction. If you say, "The cup is right behind you," she may have no idea what that means since she can't see the cup. Instead, go to her and gently turn her around so she can see it, guide her to a chair, and place the glass in her hand while you offer her a reassuring comment, "Here's your cup with your favorite juice. Come sit in this chair" (as you pat the chair). "Now you can enjoy your juice."

This step-by-step guidance may sound tedious, but it'll soon become second nature to you. The little extra time it takes to coach her will spare you a lot of aggravation that would result from Molly's confusion and frustration.

(See also: Bathroom; Choices; Compliments; Dressing; Eating; Health; Walking)

Coaching

■ ■ ■ ■ ■ ■ ■
Communication

C

When you make it a habit to routinely "talk through" your actions, you'll find that your mother is better able to give you a coherent response. If she doesn't understand something, she's apt to respond with a firm "No." That way she won't have to deal with something that she doesn't understand, and she retains her dignity and self-control. If you rephrase your comment or question and precede it with a description or elaboration, she'll have more of a chance to process your meaning before responding.

When you ask Mom, "Do you want to take a walk?" at that moment she may not be sure what "walk" means, and her response might be an emphatic "No!"

But you might get a very different reaction if you present it in another way, for example, like this: "Mom, it's so beautiful out. And it's springtime. Yesterday morning you made me promise that we'd go for a stroll around the block if the weather stayed warm. Maybe the daffodils will be in bloom in our neighbor's yard down the road. Come on, let's put on our walking shoes and go for a walk, okay?"

As much as possible, include your mother in your suggestions. Be positive and upbeat: "I promised you this." (Meaning: this is something you wished for.) Or, "This is your idea; I think it's a really good one." Or, "You asked me to remind you that you wanted to do this now. I'm so glad I remembered." Or, "This is one of your favorite things to do, isn't it?"

Because Mom has trouble expressing herself, you'll often have to think and speak out loud for her. Complete your sentences with "isn't it?" or "don't you think?" or something like that, so she will feel as if you're including her in the conversation. For example, you could say, "That was a good lunch, don't you think?" Or, "I think this is good idea, don't you agree?"

All Mom has to do is answer yes or no, and yet she will feel as though you're asking for her opinion. As you become used to this kind of communication, you'll find it much easier to deal with the more challenging situations. For example, you could say to her, "Friday's a good day for a bath, don't you think?" Or, "I'd bet you need to go to the bathroom right about now, don't you?" Or, "I'm tired and feel like going to bed, don't you?"

(*See also:* Attitude; Choices; Empathy; Normal; Questions; Validation)

■ ■ ■ ■ ■ ■ ■ ■
Compliments

Periodic sprinklings of compliments during the day will help you to keep your husband from getting restless. When he starts to become agitated, you can face him up close and, in a loving, intimate voice, say, "Have I told you lately how happy I am that we are here together? I do enjoy being with you."

Or when you're helping him get dressed, you might remember that he's been kind of moody, so you find a way to compliment him. You can say, "This shirt looks so good on you. It brings out the color in your eyes." Or, "I really like your new haircut. You look so handsome."

You can keep a repertoire of compliments handy. They can cover a lot of ground. For example, you could say things like, "You look just great in green." Or, "You've always known what to do in these kinds of situations." Or, "Thank you for suggesting this." Or, "That's a wonderful idea. I'm glad you thought of it." (Even if it was your idea.) Or, "Will you help me with this? You're so good at it." Or, "What would I do without you?" And so on.

There will be times when a simple compliment will not be enough to soothe him. You may have to take it a step further and engage him in a slightly more complex conversation to divert his attention from his agitation. Something along the lines of, "Sweetheart, do you have a moment? I really need to talk to you. It always helps me to hear what you think." And then you find some small "problem" he can help you with.

From past experiences you probably know which of your "problems" is his favorite. It doesn't matter if you have used it many times before. If you think he might remember, you can start out by saying, "I may have mentioned this to you before, but . . ."

Then, you explain your "problem" to him in great detail very seriously, and after he's given his opinion, which can be a simple yes or no, you let him know how much you value his input and opinion. You can say, "I'm so glad we talked about this. Discussing my problems with you always makes me feel so much better."

(*See also*: Affection; Dignity; Empathy; Validation)

■ ■ ■ ■ ■ ■ ■ ■
Comprehension

It's difficult to discern how much a person with dementia comprehends at any one time. It most likely varies with what else is happening at the time. Noises, crowds, the need to go the bathroom, or being hungry can all be so distracting that nothing much gets through. At other times even a nonverbal person may be able to express quite complex thoughts. It's always a good idea to assume that the person with Alzheimer's understands everything being said by you and others, even if he or she cannot give you an appropriate response.

Include your grandfather in regular conversations, and always talk to him in a normal tone of voice. If other people are involved, you may have to be proactive and repeat parts of the conversation to him while you steer the others into talking directly to him, even if he doesn't respond. Conversations provide Grandpa with important stimulation. Whether or not he comprehends doesn't matter as much as his being able to communicate his thoughts to the best of his ability.

Grandpa may seem as if he's listening with rapt attention to your account of a trip to the post office until he says, with a big grin, "All the balls are gone." This response may seem totally unrelated, but his facial expression suggests he thinks that his remark suits your conversation, so you can treat it as such because it's his participation that's important, not the words he chooses.

Of course, there will be times when it's necessary for Grandpa to really understand what you're saying: for example, when you have to give him medication, get him into the bathtub, or buckle his seat belt. In these kinds of situations, be calm while using a loving, normal adult voice. You may have to repeat your directions several times. If you start losing your patience, take a break and try again later.

(*See also:* Attitude, Communication, Empathy, Listening, Questions)

■ ■ ■ ■ ■ ■ ■
Confusion

See: Alzheimer's Disease; Choices; Communication; Conversations; Dementia; Visitors; Word Substitutions

■ ■ ■ ■ ■ ■ ■
Conversations

Conversations with an Alzheimer's person can be tricky. We don't realize how often we refer to memories in our normal small talk. This puts additional pressure on a person with memory loss. Not only may she have difficulty with the language itself, but any reference to memories can bewilder her. In the early stages of her memory loss, talk about memories can remind her of her problems, which causes unnecessary stress. However, conversations are crucial to everyone's well-being, so the trick is to have exchanges that are positive and stimulating.

You're not sure how much Mom remembers. If you talk about something specific, you may put pressure on her to remember it. However, by talking in generalities, she has the choice of a "yes" or "no" to respond to you, or she may remember something that relates. Specifics don't really matter, as long as she feels the two of you are having a conversation. You're not testing her memory as long as you stay away from "Do you remember?" Or you can put yourself in her shoes by saying, "I don't remember, do you?" Then when she answers "No," you can share a chuckle over bad memories.

By using, "don't you think?" or "weren't you?" or "wouldn't you say?" you're keeping the channels open. She may start what sounds

C

like rambling to your ear. When that happens, take a deep breath and listen to her with as much interest as you can. She's trying to let you know that she's enjoying having a real exchange with you. Remember, it's the feeling that counts and not the content. Keep your conversational tone pitched at an adult level. Your mother is not a child, so don't speak to her as if she were one. Cutesy chitchat is demeaning to both of you.

GO WITH THE FLOW
Suppose one afternoon you are listening to an "oldie," a Glenn Miller tune, with your mom. You feel like having a little conversation and you say to her: "What's the name of that? I don't remember, do you?" She might answer something like, "Harold."

Instead of repeating your question, or trying to make sense of "Harold," say, "Oh, I thought it might have been *In the Mood.*"

Your mother might respond with "I got the book." So, to keep the flow going, you might say, for example, "Do you still have it?"

To which she might respond, "I have to go home now."

So you say, "Gee Mom, we're having such a good time. Before you go anywhere, I'd like to share a bowl of strawberries with you. Isn't that a good idea?"

Your mom will be delighted because you are going with her flow and responding to her remarks, which makes her feel as if you're interested in what she says. Also you can sprinkle your conversation with occasional compliments.

Talk about something that you personally find interesting. Your attitude will rub off on her. If you choose a favorite topic that you've used before, open it with one of the following introductions. If she does by some chance remember, she will not be offended:

"I may already have told you about this . . ."

"I don't know if I told about you this, but . . ."

"This happened a long time ago, so I don't know if you'd remember . . ."

"We met so many people and did so much today, it may be hard to remember . . ."

Then you can proceed, talking to her as you would talk to a friend. She'll appreciate that you treat her as an equal adult. Since you'll be just relating your own thoughts and memories, or interesting news events, you can go on chatting away for as long as she seems interested. On the other hand, if it's important for her to understand you, slow down and enunciate clearly, repeating and rephrasing if necessary, but always using your adult tone.

WITH STRANGERS   Your mother still enjoys being part of a group, although she's no longer able to carry on a conversation in the usual sense of the word. There's no way of knowing just how much she understands, but it doesn't really matter. It's likely she hears and perceives more than we assume.

Consider this situation: Mom got all dressed up to go to a party with you. Once there, people talk to you and to each other, but your mother is not really able to participate because nobody says anything to her except for an occasional single-sentence greeting. It disturbs you that everyone ignores her, even though she's right there in their midst. People who are unfamiliar (and uncomfortable) with dementia may ignore her and talk exclusively to you, sometimes with inappropriate questions and remarks that can be disturbing or hurtful to her. For example, an acquaintance might ask you right in front of Mom: "So, she's the one with Alzheimer's, eh? Isn't she in a nursing home yet? Gee, I can't imagine how you put up with . . ."

At that point, interrupting your acquaintance is perfectly appropriate in light of her insensitivity. You can stop her in midsentence by turning to Mom as you calmly rephrase the remark and make it clear that your mother has heard every inconsiderate word: "Mom, as you can hear, this person's asking me about the tests you had done at the doctor's the other day, and she wants to know if you still live with me."

Turning to your acquaintance, you can add: "We don't have the results yet, but you know what? It doesn't really matter, because Mom and I have a good time and we're so lucky we have this time together, aren't we, Mom?"

You must assume that your mother understood the insensitive comment, so your interruption lets your acquaintance know that you consider Mom as having a part in the conversation. Hopefully, you've made it clear that such callous remarks are inappropriate. If she persists, you'll want to be more direct and stand up for Mom by saying something like this: "Your remarks are thoughtless and unkind. My mother may have dementia, but she can still hear perfectly well. Would you please change the subject?"

(*See also:* Baby Talk; Comprehension; Dignity; Normal; Validation)

■ ■ ■ ■ ■ ■ ■ ■
Counseling

Caregiving is a trying experience for most people. There are times when you're so frustrated that you think you cannot take another day. When these feelings well up in you, they're often accompanied by guilt, making you even more stressed.

Try to share these feelings with your family or your Alzheimer's Association support group as often as you can. However, sometimes it's difficult to be totally free with the group. If you find that you're unable to open up, consider professional counseling for yourself. Seeking counseling doesn't mean you're crazy, but repressing your feelings is. You need to let your feelings out, look at them, and get some help looking for solutions. A therapist can be your best ally.

A counselor or therapist can provide you with a truly safe place in which to vent all of your anger and resentment. Ask your friends for a recommendation or, if that's not comfortable, talk to your doctor about a referral. Your local hospital even may have a caregivers' support group that you can join.

Since your Dad's been living with you, you've become extraordinarily patient and quite adept at holding back your feelings. Your father has become very responsive, and you're doing well most of the time, but you've also paid a heavy price. It's as if everything's always about Dad—his needs and his comfort—while your own feelings get pushed down or to the side. You know that Dad's doing the best he can, so you feel guilty for wanting your own needs met too.

Such feelings are natural and seeking support is the healthiest thing you can do for yourself. If you're unsure about counseling, consider it something you can do that will help your father as well as you. His moods and behavior reflect yours. If you feel good, then he's calm and cooperative, but if you're upset, he will become more confused and crankier. If you can find relief somewhere, it will make life easier for both of you.

(*See also:* Depression; Family; Forgiveness; Guilt; Home Help; Respite; Stress; Support Groups)

■ ■ ■ ■ ■ ■ ■ ■
Crowds

Most of us thrive on being out in the world, but there may come a time when your Alzheimer's person can no longer handle the stimulation of crowds and noise. You don't necessarily have to discontinue your outings right away, but rather select venues that are more contained and low-key. There may come a time when going out is no longer feasible, but it's important for your person to feel a part of the world as long as possible.

Suppose you and Aunt Polly are browsing at her favorite department store. It's the big sale of the season so it's crowded and noisy. Hunting for the best sales was always the highlight of Polly's shopping excursions, so you are surprised when she becomes quite upset and pulls away from you. You can barely catch up with her as she makes a beeline for the exit. When you catch up with her, you could try to steer her instead to the shoe department, which used to keep her engrossed for hours. Say to her, "Polly, let's look over here. Maybe we'll find some new walking shoes. Look at these nice brown ones."

But when you turn to her for the enthusiastic reaction you're expecting, she looks at you with tears welling up in her eyes. You then have no choice but to spirit her out of there as quickly as you can. You can take her by the hand and gently talk to her about finding a peaceful little place to have a nice cool glass of lemonade.

Polly's probably suffering from sensory overload: too much noise, too many people, and too much going on all at once. Malls and large stores can be very bewildering for someone who has trouble sorting out impressions, so consider shopping at smaller stores and boutiques.

C

The hardest situations for Polly may be those involving relatives and friends who love her. She may feel overwhelmed at large family gatherings and react with agitation. Try to explain to everyone that Polly becomes easily unsettled by crowds and prefers one-on-one encounters. Then you can help her find a quiet corner and steer the other family members to visit with her there.

(*See also:* Attitude; Empathy; Outings; Restaurants)

■ ■ ■ ■ ■ ■ ■ ■

Cursing

It's not uncommon for someone with dementia to display behavior that has been suppressed since childhood. Cursing is one of the behaviors that may surface. When you're confronted by a sudden stream of expletives, try to remain calm and remember that it's the disease doing the talking and your father is not in control of his actions.

Your father has been in his own world all afternoon. You've tried diverting him, but he just keeps pacing up and down the hallway. He's been mumbling to himself when suddenly he lets out a loud tirade of curses, words you've never heard from him before. Over the years he'd let out an occasional "damn" or "hell" when he had a mishap, but he'd always apologize to anyone within earshot. Once he even washed your mouth out with soap when you were experimenting with creative language yourself at the age of ten. Now he's exploding with a full repertoire of curse words and you are stunned. Your first inclination may be to firmly stop him: You may want to say. "Dad! What are you saying? I don't allow that kind of talk in my house. Stop it right now!" Instead, take a deep breath and try not to react. Relax and try to make light of it by joining him in a couple of expletives:

"Motherfucker sure is a funny-sounding word, when you really listen to it, isn't it?"

You can also try humor. Ask him seriously, "Do you mean a big shithead or just a middlin' asshole?"

If you use his swear words in a normal conversation, he may hear that they're not so special and he'll become uninterested. Or you may choose to ignore his outbursts completely. This issue will have to be dealt with by trial and error. If this occurs in public, gently say to him, "Dad, this gentleman isn't familiar with that word. Maybe you can think of another word." Then turn to the stranger and let him know what's going on. Say, "This is just a phase of Alzheimer's. Please don't take it seriously."

(*See also:* Communication; Humor; Laughter)

D

■ ■ ■ ■ ■ ■ ■ ■
Day Care

There's a growing awareness of the need for stimulating and safe day care for adults who have special needs. Full-time day care can allow you to keep your job and a steady income and part-time day care can provide you with a much-deserved respite. Contact one of your state's agencies on aging for some suggestions.

You've always enjoyed your full-time job. And now that your father is living with you, you may realize that you value it even more because it helps you stay grounded and connected to the outside world. By going to work and interacting with fellow employees, customers, or clients, you experience the stimulation, personal connection, and emotional support that create a healthy balance in your own life. When you return home to your father you're more likely to feel renewed and recharged.

Your dad used to be fine at home on his own but, lately, that seems to have changed. Sometimes he's withdrawn and depressed by the time you get back from work. If you ask him what he had for lunch, he may be so vague that you suspect he hasn't eaten a thing. At that point, you may realize that he can't be left alone anymore, and that you need help looking after him while you're at work.

Some of the options open to you are home care, adult day care, or a senior center. At this point, adult day care seems to be the ideal solution, because it offers your father both social interaction and mental stimulation. Because it's too difficult for him to entertain himself now, and he's too forgetful to take care of his own meals, adult day care would provide a remedy for both of these concerns.

When you return home at the end of your workday, share an amusing or exciting anecdote with your father. If you had a dull day, make something up or retell an old favorite incident of his. Your father may not be able to give you feedback, but continue talking for as long as he appears to be interested. He will appreciate that you consider him important enough to want to share your daily experiences with him.

(*See also:* Home Help; Respite; Share Care; Support Groups)

D

■■■■■■■■
Death and Dying

It's likely that you'll be involved with your father's final departure from this world. This is really hard for most of us to face and we tend to postpone thinking about it. If you can concentrate on wanting to make his passing the best possible experience for him, it might help you. There's help and support out there for you. Hospice programs offer help to you and your father. You might want to talk to your local chapter now about some of the details.

Imagine that many mourners are gathered around the casket at the graveside of an old and dear friend of your father's. More people are still making their way across the grass. You and your father have been standing there for a while, when he suddenly asks very loudly, "When's the train coming?" Heads turn and you become embarrassed.

It is such a somber group, mostly strangers who don't know about your dad's dementia. You must admit that the crowd does look like a bunch of commuters waiting for the 5:24 express. Quietly explain to your father that this is not a train platform but rather a funeral for his friend John. He seems to accept your explanation and watches the late arrivals in silence for a while. Surveying the crowd, he says, "No wonder John's not here. He's such a happy person and everyone here is so sad."

At that point, you might decide that Dad doesn't really grasp what's happening and you know that he doesn't need to be exposed to any more sadness, so you lead him back to the car. While you are stuck in the lineup of parked cars, take the opportunity to talk to your father about his own wishes. "That was an awfully serious service. It sounded to me as if you think John would have liked something different. How about *your* celebration? What would you like?"

Your father flashes you a big grin and says, "I want everyone to have a good time with happy music, good food, chocolate ice cream, and lots of funny stories."

D

Although you've always known it was inevitable, the thought of your father's death has always depressed you. The two of you have never talked about it until now, yet under the circumstances it may seem easy. Tell him, "I promise we'll have a great party for you. But I must tell you, Dad, that I'll still be sad, because I'll miss you very much. However, we don't have to talk about it for a long time, thank goodness. As soon as we can get out of here, let's go and test some ice creams, okay?"

Fill the rest of your wait in the car talking about the trees and flowers around you and other unrelated topics. Most likely your father will have completely forgotten why he's there. As you contemplate your conversation, make a silent vow to yourself to try to make each day with your father worth remembering.

You've spent the last months or years making a wonderful life for your mother. You've shared joys and laughter with her and you've filled her life with many special experiences. Recently, however, she's become quite weak and withdrawn. You suspect that her end might be near. You're hoping that she'll go quietly in her sleep in her own bed, just as she has always wanted.

However, the final episode may include having to take her to the hospital. If she's terminally ill and there's nothing more that medicine can do for her, then you have two options: to let her life wind down naturally or to keep her on life support indefinitely. Be sure to have her living will in place. This will states her last wishes. If she does not want to have life support once she reaches a terminal stage, then you must decide if you want her to die in a hospital or at home, where you can keep her comfortable in her own bed and in her own surroundings. A social worker at the hospital can put you in touch with hospice or home-care personnel who can help with her care at home. A hospice can also help you with pain control if that's necessary.

Death and Dying

Keep her environment and routines as normal as possible. Even if your mother is comatose, you can still read to her or talk to her while playing soothing music in the background. This would be easy to do at home, but at the hospital you may need to bring a small cassette or CD player with headphones so she can listen to her favorite music. It's a well-recognized fact that the awareness of music is the last sensation to go. Also, music will drown out hospital noises and help create a peaceful environment.

Whether your mom's at home or in the hospital, talk to her in your normal, gentle voice. If she's at all aware, she will need to hear that you're there with her. It might be very difficult for you, but try not to let your own fears and grief show. Your mother may be aware of her own impending death, so let her know that you're aware as well. One approach might be: "Mom, I love you and I'll miss you a lot, but it's okay for you to leave anytime you wish. We're okay and we can take care of everything."

If she's able to talk, she may need to express her fears and anxieties. As good as you are at communicating with her, this will be the toughest test for you yet. You need to be your mother's pillar of strength at a time when you yourself are likely to be devastated with grief. She will also need to feel your touch; so hold her hand as much as possible and give her a gentle back rub or foot massage. If she's comatose, hold her hand or rub her arms. Then you might gently say to her: "I love you, Mom. Everything's been taken care of. It's all right for you to rest now."

And if she's religious, you can add, "The angels are waiting for you, Mom. God loves you and I love you."

> **Tip!** Final arrangements are much easier to deal with ahead of time. Confer with several mortuaries about costs and arrangements so you won't be forced to make decisions while you are in an emotionally distraught state. Be sure that you've already talked to your mother about her last wishes, especially regarding cremation. Ask her doctor to instruct you on the procedures you can expect at the time of her death.

(See also: Affection; Dignity; Empathy; Massage; Normal; Paperwork)

Death and Dying

■■■■■■■■
Dementia

Dementia is an umbrella term used to describe conditions that exhibit memory loss and confusion. There are dozens of causes of dementia aside from Alzheimer's, including many that may be correctable, such as hypothyroidism, normal pressure hydrocephalus, and vitamin deficiencies (Crystal et al. 2000). Sometimes it's hard to distinguish dementia from what doctors call *delirium*, or severe confusion due to illness. Delirium is reversible and may be caused by dehydration, pneumonia, drug reactions, or a severe exacerbation of many preexisting conditions. Personality changes are occasionally the first symptom of brain tumors.

> **Alzheimer's disease** is the most common irreversible dementia. The other two most prevalent dementias are Lewy body dementia and vascular or multi-infarct dementia.

> **Lewy body dementia** is closely related to Parkinson's disease and may coexist with that. Rigidity and difficulty initiating movement along with severe hallucinations, delusions, and aggressive outbursts usually appear before real memory loss becomes apparent. It's quite difficult to distinguish from Alzheimer's and it may benefit from some of the same therapy (Ballard, Grace, and Holmes 1998).

> **Vascular dementia** is the broad term for dementia associated with problems with the circulation of blood to the brain. It can be caused by high blood pressure, high cholesterol, and strokes. *Multi-infarct dementia* is caused by repeated strokes, which can either be several large strokes or a combination of strokes of varying severity. *Transient ischemic attacks (TIAs)* cause temporary neurological deficits and are a warning that a stroke may occur soon or that small "ministrokes" could occur or are occurring. Your doctor should be informed if these are occurring (de la Torre 2004).

> **Frontal lobe dementia** is the name given to any dementia caused by damage to this part of the brain. It includes

Pick's disease, but can also be caused by genetic predisposition and other diseases. The frontal lobe governs mood, behavior, and self-control. Damage leads to changes in the way a person feels and expresses emotion, and to loss of judgment (Mendonça et al. 2004).

Alcohol-related dementia is caused by excessive use of alcohol (Mukama et al. 2003). It's usually also related to a deficiency in thiamine and vitamin B_1. Initial symptoms are similar to those of early Alzheimer's disease, but they may be improved or reversed with vitamin therapy.

It's important to distinguish between normal "senior moments," like forgetting your grandchild's name, and more serious lapses, like forgetting that you have a family. Periodic memory lapses are normal. Our brains will retain and supply facts quickly as long as there's a natural connection to something else currently appearing in a thought train. In other words, it's harder for any of us to remember something that is completely unrelated. As we become older, our brains have so much more to sort through to recollect a specific thought that recall may be much slower; but this is not Alzheimer's disease.

Your aunt always kept track of everyone's birthday and anniversary, calling the rest of you to remind you to send a card or a bouquet of flowers. She used to be so sure of herself; she was outgoing and quick to break into a smile. Lately things have been different. This woman, who was once known as an impeccable fashion plate, now often dresses in inappropriate outfits and has even shown up disheveled at family gatherings. She is becoming withdrawn and anxious and will break into tears at the smallest upset. Your aunt, who was the keeper of the family archives, now has trouble remembering the names of her own children and sometimes will even furiously deny that she has any nieces and nephews.

You fear that your aunt may be developing Alzheimer's disease. But before you jump to this conclusion, keep in mind that many people develop dementia from disorders that may be reversible. It's important for her to see a doctor for a thorough physical and for mental testing. After all else has been eliminated, the probable diagnosis may, in fact, be Alzheimer's. There's a real advantage to knowing this

Dementia

as early as possible. Your aunt can get started on one of the Alzheimer's medications and she can participate in planning for her future.

If your aunt's dementia has come on suddenly, you'll want her to see her doctor immediately. It could be a reaction to an infection or a nutritional deficiency. Bring a complete list of her food and drug intake with you, including prescriptions, over-the-counter medications, vitamins, and alternative supplements. Your aunt should have thorough physical examinations, including MRIs and CAT scans, which are particularly good for detecting brain tumors, fluid on the brain, and blood clots. Request extensive blood tests and discuss tests for possible food allergies.

(*See also:* Alternative Remedies; Alzheimer's Disease; Alzheimer's Medications; Diet and Nutrition; Health; Vitamins)

■ ■ ■ ■ ■ ■ ■ ■
Dental Health

Toothaches, gum disease, and other dental problems can aggravate Alzheimer's disease. It's a good idea to take your uncle for a cleaning and checkup every three to four months. His dentist may be able to catch cavities before they become a serious problem. A toothache can be serious for your uncle. It can cause eating problems and lead to infections of the gums. He may also experience pain that he is not able to convey to you.

Your uncle doesn't want to brush his teeth. He may be reluctant because he's forgotten how to use toothpaste or he may even have difficulty with the brushing itself. Try making it a shared experience by brushing your own teeth at the same time. Chat about how he taught you to brush correctly, which will allow you to casually demonstrate for him, "This is how you showed me when I was a little kid. I still brush exactly the same way, see?"

If you think your uncle may be swallowing the toothpaste, you can apply a very small dab of the paste to his wet brush, just enough to add a little flavor. You may even leave out the paste altogether, because it's the brushing itself that's important. Use a soft bristle brush, possibly a child's size if that will help him reach back to his molars. It's a good idea to soak his brush overnight in a mixture of half water and half peroxide to kill germs.

When your uncle can no longer brush by himself, you'll have to do it for him. Have him sit in a low chair so you can comfortably stand behind him, and cup his chin in one hand while you brush his teeth with your other hand. You'll want to make sure that his gums get massaged well and, if he'll let you, you can floss his teeth as well. It may take a few tries before you're both comfortable with this new routine. To help him feel safer, talk to him and explain what you're doing and why. Use a light, positive tone and you can even joke about your own awkwardness, since this is new to both of you.

If you're not sure how to go about this, ask his dentist to demonstrate for you. Having his dentist involved makes it easier for you to tell him honestly that these are his doctor's orders, even if he doesn't remember.

DENTURES   If your father wears dentures, you should check his gums periodically. Red spots can develop from irritation caused by food particles that have worked their way under his plate, making his gums tender. The spots also may result from a bad fit, causing the dentures to rub against his gums. Speak to his dentist for advice about this problem.

(See also: Body Language; Communication; Health; Vitamins)

■ ■ ■ ■ ■ ■ ■ ■

Depression

Sometimes your sister will burst into tears without any obvious provocation. She may be suffering from depression. It may stem from her feeling useless and out of place. You can talk until you're blue in the face about how much you love her and want her to live with you, but it won't help until your sister regains some sort of self-respect and feels like a functioning member of society again. Let her know that you need her help. Be sincere, because if you gush too much, all of your good intentions could backfire, and she might feel ridiculed and further alienated.

Using suggestions in this book as a guideline, design a few activities specifically tailored to your sister's interests. Start slowly with a small project and build it up as she responds. Your first projects should help her to feel useful again. Ask her honestly for her opinions and her suggestions and always listen patiently to her reply, even if you don't really understand it.

If you've tried every approach outlined in this book and she still doesn't respond, it may be time to seek professional help for her. Antidepressant drugs available by prescription seem to benefit many Alzheimer's people by relieving anxiety and lifting the spirits. There are also antidepressant herbal and homeopathic remedies available, but before you make a choice, be sure to confer with a health professional. There can be unpleasant side effects and interactions with any medication, whether prescription or over-the-counter. Keep a journal of your sister's emotional state, attitude, and spirit.

(*See also:* Activities; Alternative Remedies; Diversions; Health; Humor; Laughter)

■ ■ ■ ■ ■ ■ ■ ■
Diet and Nutrition

Many elderly folks just don't eat enough and often develop vitamin deficiencies. Malnutrition, dehydration, and vitamin deficiencies are often found in those suffering from cognitive disorders, such as Alzheimer's disease. Some of these deficiencies are reversible, but even if the damage has already been done, it doesn't hurt to do everything in your power to slow down further deterioration. Regardless of the cause of your mother's dementia, you can help her enormously by making some changes in her diet (Weil 1998). You'll want to eliminate foods high in saturated fats and sugar, both of which may aggravate dementia. Next, talk to her doctor about putting her on a strong multivitamin with minerals and adding extra amounts of vitamins E and C.

You'll want to avoid processed foods, white flour products, sugar, food coloring, and hydrogenated oil products (margarine) which contain trans-fatty acids. The healthy diet for your mother and any one of us is built around fresh seasonal vegetables and fruits, and whole grain cereals and breads. Lean red meats and fatty fish, dairy products (if tolerated), and olive or canola oil are also good foods for people with dementia.

Leafy vegetables, red onions, fresh citrus fruit, and even coffee are high in bioflavonoids, which are antioxidants that support the work that vitamin C does. Recently, bioflavonoids have been found to lower cholesterol as well.

Carrots, squash, sweet potatoes, and cantaloupe are good foods. So are pink grapefruit and tomatoes. Any fruits or vegetables with an orange or red hue are good sources of beta-carotene. Beta-carotene converts into vitamin A, which is essential for cell growth and development. Dark green leafy vegetables also provide beta-carotene.

Canola oil, flaxseed oil, walnuts, fatty fish (sardines, herring, swordfish, and salmon) are also good foods. Polyunsaturated fats, also known as Omega-3 fatty acids, prevent heart disease and fight cancer (Dixon and Ernst 2001).

Soybeans, tofu, soy milk, lentils, chickpeas, and kidney beans are excellent sources of isoflavones, which provide estrogen-like compounds when estrogen is low, and they also provide protection against breast cancer (Biermann 2002).

Water is very important. Elderly folks in general are notoriously conservative in their liquid intake. Your mother's generation considered water something you used to swallow your medication or to rinse with after brushing your teeth. They must find the current preoccupation with designer waters puzzling. Keeping that in mind, if your mother resists drinking plain water, you can create refreshing and healthy "ades." Mix frozen juice with twice the amount of water suggested on the can and add sweetener to taste. The goal is for your Alzheimer's person to drink eight glasses of water a day.

Alcohol. Alcohol impairs everyone's ability to think clearly, and for people with Alzheimer's, its effect is amplified. You probably should not give an Alzheimer's patient more than one drink per day. Excessive use of alcohol has been linked to the development of Alzheimer's disease (Mukamal et al. 2003).

Smoothies are very good. If your mother has trouble eating, you can make delicious smoothies for her and add all kinds of healthy things. Use a base of yogurt, fruit juice, or soy, rice, or whey milk. Then add one or several goodies like lecithin, an Omega-3 oil like flaxseed oil, bee pollen, soy protein, powdered gelatin, or nutritional yeast. Whip up the mixture in a blender with a banana or other fruits. If you need to, you can sweeten it with honey or flavor it with vanilla. Most health food stores have nutritional specialists who can advise you and give you recipes.

(*See also:* Alternative Remedies; Alzheimer's Disease; Vitamins)

■ ■ ■ ■ ■ ■ ■ ■
Dignity

Your mother needs you to become the guardian of her self-respect and dignity, especially as her confusion increases. You'll speak out on her behalf in ways you never would have imagined. It may have taken you a while to build up your nerve, but now you interrupt others who insist on talking to her in a patronizing tone, and you stop people who speak about your mother as if she wasn't there. Your mom may not be able to let you know in words how much she appreciates your interventions on her behalf, but her behavior will tell you.

Imagine you and your mother are having a lovely lunch at your favorite restaurant when she suddenly gets a funny, distracted look on her face. You ask her if she likes the food and she mumbles that it's really good, so that's not the reason for her expression. Then you ask her if she needs the toilet, but she shakes her head no. Then you happen to notice the tag of her tea bag hanging out on the side of her mouth. You reach across the table and gently remove the tea bag with a napkin. She's already bitten into it and her mouth is full of loose tea, so you say to her: "That doesn't taste very good, does it? Go ahead and spit out the rest of it in this napkin and then you can rinse out your mouth with some water."

The people sitting at the table next to yours have witnessed this and are staring at you, but you ignore them and continue to help your mother spit the tea leaves out into the water glass and you ask the waiter for a fresh glass of water. This has never happened before and you are a little shaken, but by treating this as if it's a perfectly normal occurrence, you will help your mother maintain her dignity and good spirits. After she rinses out her mouth she will quickly forget about the whole incident and will continue eating her meal.

D

Your family considered eating out to be a special occasion. Your mother still gets excited about going out to a restaurant. You aren't going to let the tea bag episode stop you from taking her out, but you will want to avoid this kind of embarrassment in the future. So, the next time you are at a restaurant, you might want to hold her drink for her, so she won't confuse it with her solid foods. You also can ask the waiter to arrange a special plate for her. It may be easier for her if she has only one kind of food at a time, either all finger food or all fork food.

At times, it will be quite a task to maintain your mother's dignity, but with your positive attitude and relaxed approach you'll manage to get through these moments by reminding yourself that no one ever died from embarrassment.

(*See also:* Affection; Attitude; Body Language; Compliments; Validation)

■ ■ ■ ■ ■ ■ ■ ■
Discussions

Your wife has always been intrigued by science, history, and anything else based in fact. You watch PBS and the Discovery Channel with her and you read to her from *Scientific American*, *Nature*, and *National Geographic*. Although she's not really able to discuss much with you, she never takes her eyes off you whenever you read to her. Even when you read the same thing for the tenth time, try to approach it as if it were the first time and read it with the enthusiasm and gusto of discovery: "Listen to this, Hon. I found a really provocative article. I can't wait to share it with you. I'll bet you'll like it; I found it very interesting. Would you like to hear it right now?" Since you've read it to her before, there's a chance that she'll interact with you so you can stimulate a discussion by sharing ideas with her.

———————

Serious adult discussions are as important to your father as they are to you, even if he's not able to contribute much anymore. Think about what you talk about with your friends and try to discuss the same subjects with him. You can talk about a topic you know he's interested in or you can consult with him about something happening in your personal life. For example, you might say, "Dad, I could really use your advice on something important to me. I'm considering moving my office at work. Tell me what you think, okay? My office now has a good view but very cramped space. I can move into a bigger space but it has no windows. What would be important to you, more space or a view?"

Give him enough time to react to your question. If he responds with a totally unrelated remark, go with his flow, no matter where it goes. You may have to slow down and simplify your choice of words, but talk to him like an adult, and avoid using a condescending tone. Engaging in adult conversations helps your father maintain his self-esteem and dignity, even if his responses are incoherent or disjointed.

(See also: Communication; Conversations; Listening; Normal; Questions; Validation)

■ ■ ■ ■ ■ ■ ■ ■
Diversions

Grandma has been living with you for the last couple of years. Every so often she becomes obsessed with wanting to "go home." She stands at the front door in her overcoat, with a pair of bedroom slippers in her hand, and announces, "I'm going home now!" Then she starts to turn the door handle. You quickly go to her side, put your arm around her shoulder, and say, "Okay. I'm so sorry you have to leave so soon, Grandma, because we were having such a good visit.

Oh, I almost forgot something. I promised to show you my new earrings. Come, let me show them to you before you go."

Your grandma loves jewelry, so she gladly follows as you retrieve your jewelry box. Sit her down at the kitchen table with the box in front of her as you slip off her coat and say, "Let me take that, it's too hot in here for a coat, isn't it? I'll hang it up in the closet for you. And let's set your slippers in the closet by your coat, then you'll know where they are, okay?"

Pull out a pair of earrings for her to finger. It will be only a short time before she settles in with the entire contents of your jewelry box laid out on the kitchen table, arranging earrings in matching pairs. While you talk to her about some of the pieces, she will become so totally engrossed in all the glitter in front of her that she will forget about wanting to leave. In this way, you won't argue with her about wanting to go home; instead you've diverted her attention. You change her mind by changing her environment, and you also wind up sharing some special time with her as well.

Your father's restless and irritated. He's started pacing and mumbling angrily to himself. You've tried offering him his favorite tea, but he didn't want any. You leave the room and come back with today's mail as you say, "Dad, I'm really busy right now and I sure could use your help. Would you mind opening the mail?"

Hand him a blunt letter opener. When he cheerfully starts opening the mail, you can add, "And while you're at it, would you mind sorting it? It would be great if you'd put all the bills in one stack and the rest in another stack. I'd really appreciate your help. You've always been so much better than me at sorting things."

You might find this such a successful diversion that you can use it as a daily activity.

(*See also:* Activities; Compliments; Normal; Personal
Space; Projects; Reality; Validation)

■ ■ ■ ■ ■ ■ ■ ■

Dressing

D

Your mother wants to continue to dress herself for as long as she is able, although you'll want to keep an eye on her to make sure she dresses somewhat appropriately. She may need some assistance with which is the front or back of a dress, or which shoe goes on which foot. She may have trouble with "left and right," so use "this one" and "the other" instead.

"This shoe goes on this foot" (as you pat her leg). "Then you put the other one on the other foot. There you are, ready to walk!"

If your mother still selects her own wardrobe, she may forget that she wore the same outfit yesterday. Perhaps she chose it because it's hanging right there in the front of the closet or maybe because it's her favorite dress. To discourage her from picking the same clothes all the time, go to her closet when she's not in her room and remove the often-worn outfit so that it's not available the next morning for her to wear. If that doesn't work, the next time she reaches for the same old dress, distract her by offering her another one. "How about this blue dress, Mom? You look so pretty in blue. It makes your eyes shine."

Suppose the two of you have been invited to lunch at a friend's house and your mother has been in her room getting dressed. After forty-five minutes you decide to check on her. She beams at you as she says, "I'm almost ready!" She's wearing three skirts on top of her slacks, along with two scarves. First take a deep breath, then say, "Wow, that certainly is a creative outfit you've got on. But, you know what, it's kind of hot today. I think you'll roast in all of those clothes. How about choosing just one outfit? I like the skirt with the flowers. It goes so well with your blouse. Let me help you."

Getting dressed can be a confusing experience. Panties have three openings and your mother may not be able to discern into which opening to place her foot. A dress also can be a nightmare, and it's easy for your mother to become tangled in a full skirt. She may need a guiding hand from you. When you help her, keep it dignified and talk about how you experience similar problems with your own clothes.

Buy Mom attractive garments that are comfortable, nonbinding, and one size too large. Have your mother wear socks instead of stockings, and buy loose-fitting queen-size knee-high nylons that won't cut off her circulation, in case she must attend an event where wearing hosiery is an absolute necessity.

Use undershirts instead of brassieres. Your mother may find a turtleneck uncomfortable; instead choose a boatneck, crewneck, or cowl neck. If she often undresses in public, clothe her in outfits that button or zip in the back. Bring extra clothes with you in the car: a change of pants, a sweater, a top, and extra pads.

MAKEUP   You help your mother with bathing and brushing her teeth. You comb her hair and watch her discreetly while she dresses. She has always worn makeup and still tries to apply her own lipstick, at times with interesting results. Her favorite color is bright red, which she shakily applies to chin and cheeks as well as to her lips. Looking at herself in the mirror, she may seem satisfied with her appearance and you've learned to live with it.

This is not a problem at home, but when you go out in public, your mother often draws startled glances from strangers. You've become very good at ignoring the puzzled looks, but one day at church, the stares are so obvious that your mother becomes confused and uncomfortable.

The next day, the two of you visit your local department store makeup counter. You distract Mom by having her browse through scarves and handbags while you have a quick conference with the salesperson. When your mother eventually sits for her "makeover," the salesperson makes a big point of using a nearly colorless lip gloss. She touts it as the latest fashion while complimenting your mother on how beautiful she looks with the new color. Discard her fire-engine red lipstick when you get home. Your mother can now apply the lip gloss anywhere she wants with no visible trace. You may have to wear colorless lip gloss yourself in your mother's presence and reserve your red lipsticks for evenings out.

SHAVING   Your father has used a straight razor all his life with great macho pride, but there's no way he can use one safely now.

You've tried to convince him that wearing a beard is very manly, but even you have to admit he looks kind of shaggy. Every time you've suggested a regular razor, he protests, and besides, you're worried that he could still hurt himself. You can ask for help from a male friend of his or yours to talk to him about how masculine "new" electric razors are. At first, he may be reluctant, but the friend can probably convince him that it's completely manly. Then he can shave himself for hours on end, sometimes driving you crazy with the noise, but it will be worth it considering his clean look and the fact that he won't have lopped off any ears yet.

(*See also:* Coaching; Compliments; Dignity; Obsessive Behavior; Undressing)

■ ■ ■ ■ ■ ■ ■ ■
Driving

Giving up the car is probably the most traumatic experience an elderly person might have to undergo. Someone with early Alzheimer's may still be able to drive on familiar routes, but as the dementia progresses, the day will come when he must give it up, for his own safety and that of others on the road. It's almost never easy.

Your father's still driving, though not quite like the old days when he practically lived in his car. Usually he does well, but lately he's been missing a lot of turns and he has trouble reading road signs. Recently he was driving the two of you down the freeway when he missed your turnoff. Without thinking, you exclaimed, "Oh Dad, that was our exit! You missed it!" He stopped the car cold, put it into reverse, and backed up, oblivious to the rest of the traffic behind him.

When you got there, home never looked so good to you before. You stumbled up the front steps on your Jell-O knees, thanking every deity you could think of, and pledging to them all that this was the last time your father would ever drive again.

Boy, that's easier said than done! Your father loves his automobile with a passion. It's his pride and joy, and a symbol of his freedom. Losing his car will break his heart. You've tried to discuss the

D

subject with him before, and your otherwise gentle father hit the roof and wanted to hear nothing more about it. But since the freeway incident you've made up all kinds of excuses about why he should allow you to drive. You've tried to take his keys away, and you've even disconnected the battery. These actions kept him from driving, but Dad's becoming obsessed with his car and is suspicious when you tell him the car isn't working.

He grumbles angrily, "You just don't know anything about cars and that mechanic of yours doesn't know what he's doing."

Suppose your Dad's best friend offers to help. While you are telling him about the incident on the freeway, your father emphatically states that he would never do anything of the sort. You know that there's no point in arguing, so you take a deep breath and say instead, "Dad, you are a very good driver, but I'm worried about you when you have trouble reading the signs. I love you and I wouldn't want anything to happen to you."

This calms him down and his friend suggests a gradual tapering off. Reluctantly your father agrees that he'll only drive the two of you to your weekly visits to his sister, using a side street route he "knows" like the back of his hand, and to a couple of shops that are just around the corner. You promise not to overreact as you did on the freeway and say that from now on you'll gently guide him to the next turn without sounding too much like a backseat driver; for example, you could say, "Let's take the next turn. That'll get us to the right street."

You want to help him stay focused and calm. You won't mention missed turns. That would only aggravate him and most likely make his driving even more frightening.

When the time comes, you can ask his doctor to give Dad an official "medical order" requiring him to give up the car keys. Contact your local Alzheimer's Association for advice and guidance if you anticipate difficulties. You'll also want to encourage your dad to talk to others who have had to give up driving, so he won't feel so alone. Your local senior center may also be a good source for help with driving issues.

(*See also:* Independencce)

E

■ ■ ■ ■ ■ ■ ■ ■

Eating

Mealtimes can be the best of times or the worst for Alzheimer's people. Many will need to have several small servings throughout the day, while others do fine with a normal routine of three meals a day. Some people will suddenly become confused at the selections that are presented to them or forget how to use the utensils. Most people, even those with advanced dementia, have personal likes and dislikes for different foods and appreciate having choices. For example, Harold may be in late stage Alzheimer's and nonverbal, but he's probably able to let you know his preferences with a nod when you present them to him as two choices.

Dining is the highlight of Harold's day. He carefully tucks his napkin in at his throat or at least he makes a good attempt at it. His mother was a stickler about manners. Most of the time meals go well, but there are times when he appears confused. He'll stare at his plate and the utensils, apparently uncertain of how to get the food into his mouth. You can help him by placing the fork in his hand and closing his fingers around it. Say, "Harold, this is your favorite. It looks good, doesn't it? Here, you can use this fork to eat it."

Get into the habit of having only one utensil available at a time, which seems to help. Precut his food into bite-size pieces and arrange them on his plate to look appetizing. Also, his beverage sometimes confuses him. He may try to "eat" it with his fork or pour it over his dinner. Gently take the drink out of his hand as you say, "I'd be glad to hold your drink for you while you eat, okay?" Then, fix him a fresh plate and keep his drink separate, or hold his fork while he takes a sip of his drink.

Make sure that you don't mix foods needing different approaches on his plate. Serve only fork food or only finger food. If his hands have forgotten how to hold a sandwich, you can cut it up to become fork food. If you're eating at a restaurant, ask to have the contents of the sandwich served on a plate as separate items.

There may come a time when handling a utensil becomes too confusing for Harold. At that point you can change his diet to finger food exclusively. This may be a challenge, but it can also be interesting for you to create a well-rounded meal of finger food, such as steamed chunks of vegetables, bite-size pieces of chicken, and small pieces of fruit.

E

You used to be amazed at your mother's self-control. She'd eat so little at dinner you wondered how it was that you missed out on those thin genes. Now that she's living with you, however, you're growing concerned that she's getting too thin. She takes tiny little bites and chews each one forever.

Whenever you finished with your own meal, you'd routinely ask her, "Are you finished with your dinner?" To which she always answered, "Yes." Then one night, by chance, you phrased your question differently and asked instead, "Mom, are you still eating your dinner?" to which she responded, "Yes."

It took her forever to finish what was on her plate. An hour later, you finally cleared the table. Then it dawned on you that she's probably always been a very slow eater and, in the past, she would just automatically stop eating as soon as everyone else did, even if she was still hungry.

Now, you routinely ask her "Are you still eating?" rather than "Have you finished?" and you allot enough time for her to eat. She's started to put some weight back on her bones, which makes the extra time spent on eating worthwhile.

(*See also:* Body Language; Choices; Coaching)

E

■ ■ ■ ■ ■ ■ ■ ■
Emergency Pack

You'll want to carry an "emergency" pack with you in the car. It should contain the following:

> A standard first-aid kit

> Important papers

> Phone numbers, including medical emergency numbers

> Extra clothing: sweater, pants, and underpants

> Several panty liners, briefs (adult diapers), and an underpad

> Tissues, packaged wet towels, lotion, and sunscreen

> Entertainment and diversions: a favorite book or magazine, a word game book, a songbook, a joke book, peppermints, or crackers

> In winter, extra scarves, gloves, leggings

(*See also:* Incontinence; Paperwork)

■ ■ ■ ■ ■ ■ ■ ■
Empathy

You'll be more effective in handling Aunt Elsie's problem situations if you can empathize with her by looking at circumstances through her eyes. Learn to share her reality, even when it's very different from yours. How would it feel to be in her shoes?

How does her dementia feel to her? Picture yourself frantically searching for your car keys, but not being able to remember where you left them. Now imagine that you've finally found them, only to discover that you have absolutely no idea what you're supposed to do with them, or even what they are.

Can you imagine what it would feel like to experience that sort of confusion every single day? In your own mind you are still the same person you've always been. You still think of yourself as normal, but the world around you seems to be changing. You try to explain your dilemma to a familiar-looking person, but the words just won't come out right. You feel as if you're going crazy and start to panic. Then the familiar person looks at you with gentle eyes and says, "May I have a hug, please, Auntie?"

E

You let her hold you as calmness washes over you. You even giggle. Maybe you're not losing your mind after all. Slowly that familiar-looking person becomes recognizable: it's your niece!

Other people, however, are starting to treat you strangely. One person may pat you on the head as if you were a dog, while another coos in your face as if you were a baby. People are starting to ignore you and, even worse, they talk through you, as if you weren't even there. Your feelings haven't changed; you still feel joy, pain, longings, and love. Doesn't anybody see?

As Elsie loses her ability to communicate, it might feel to her as if she were a stranger in a foreign country, ignorant of the local language and customs. She tries to explain that she needs help, but as hard as she tries, no one seems to understand.

You're learning to be empathetic with your aunt and look at the world from her point of view. It helps you gain an understanding of her feelings, but there are still times when she catches you off guard. One day, you're surprised to find Elsie dissolving into tears. You have no idea why. When you ask, she utters forlornly, "They all left without me." You ask, "Who left without you and where are they going, Aunt Elsie?" And she responds, "They're going to the service. My sister could've waited for me. How could she do that to me?"

Comfort your aunt while you review your family history to recall any event that could have triggered such an emotional reaction. Then it hits you! Elsie's reliving her beloved grandmother's death, when she had been left at home during the funeral. You need to find a way to soothe this heartbroken ten-year-old child. Say something like, "I'm so sorry that they didn't take you, Elsie. I didn't get to go either. Come with me and we'll light a candle for Granny."

Empathy

When you "go into the space" with her, your empathy will help you to understand and share her feelings so that you can deal more effectively with all kinds of situations.

(*See also:* Attitude; Coaching; Comprehension; Normal; Reality; Validation)

E

■ ■ ■ ■ ■ ■ ■ ■

Environment

As Dad becomes more confused, his environment becomes increasingly important to him. As tempting as it might be to give a fresh new look to his room or apartment, resist the urge. If you have to move him into another space or room, try to duplicate the furnishings of his former room. He needs the psychological comfort of his favorite chair being in its usual spot in front of the chest on which all the family pictures are positioned in their familiar places. If you must make changes, do so gradually.

Your father's toy car has been with him since he was six years old, although it has little paint left after so many years of handling. As a matter of fact, you even played with it when you were small. Now it sits between the portraits of his parents and your baby picture. You carefully dust around them because your father has a fit if he thinks they've been moved. They're all in perfect view from his favorite old easy chair, which, like the toy car, is an antique of indeterminable age and indistinguishable color. You've tried in vain to convince him that he needs a replacement. You can introduce his new recliner in place of the old monstrosity by keeping a throw blanket on the old one for a few weeks, then transfer the blanket onto the new recliner, which should be positioned in exactly the same location as the old one.

(*See also:* Privacy; Signs; Transitions)

■ ■ ■ ■ ■ ■ ■ ■

Exercise

Exercise is critical to the mental and physical well-being of everybody, including Alzheimer's people. Your grandfather needs to move his body. Try to get him to raise his arms above his head and swing them back and forth. Unless he's wheelchair-bound, have him walk with you with as much vigor as he can safely handle.

E

You can also make up your own versions of exercises for Grandpa. How about taking him for a barefoot walk on the lawn in the backyard or the shoreline of the beach? Throw your arms up to the sky and make noises: oinks, moos, caws, and hollers. Challenge him to a lion-roaring contest. It's a wonderful feeling to let it all out, and it happens to be good exercise for him. You might want to borrow a child or two to help you out. Most of us adults are a little self-conscious and need practice to feel free and loose again.

DANCING   If your mother is somewhat agile and mobile, you can reintroduce her to the fine art of dancing. It's been a while since she last danced, so start slowly, watching her balance and avoiding turns or spins. Stay in one spot on the dance floor and move your arms and upper body to the music. When Mom joins in, simply synchronize your movements to hers. If she's reluctant, grasp her hands lightly and move them to the music. If she hasn't danced in a long time, it may take her a while to get back into the swing of it. Keep it light and spontaneous as you improvise your dance movements to her favorite music, whether she loves Puccini, Tommy Dorsey, or Garth Brooks.

Suppose you're playing one of Mom's favorite operas, *Madame Butterfly*. The music never fails to inspire her. She smiles and her eyes begin to shine as she starts swaying to the music. Move your chair so that you face her chair and begin moving your arms in concert with hers. At first, you both may be a little shy about your movements, but soon the two of you will be doing ballet with your upper bodies. It's so much fun that by the time the music stops you're both breathless but probably laughing because of the sheer joy the two of you have shared. Also, if your mother has serious problems with her speech, or if she is nonverbal, these movement explorations can give her a meaningful outlet for self-expression.

SWIMMING   For years your favorite exercise has been swimming, so after Grandpa moved in with you, he'd join you at the local pool. He's a strong swimmer, or at least he was. Lately you've noticed he hesitates in the middle of his familiar strokes, as though his body has forgotten these very basic moves. Your grandfather's not aware of these changes and when you point them out to him he may get quite upset.

Before he has an episode that could endanger his life, introduce him to water aerobics, exercises that can be done in the shallow end of the pool. Also, your granddad should wear a swim vest that will keep him afloat.

WALKS   Your father enjoys taking walks around the block with you. If his eyesight is good enough, you can take the time to look at all the little details along the way: a budding rose bush, a newly painted wall, or an ant colony. Later on you can recollect your adventures and tell each other, "It sure is a beautiful day today and we had a great walk, didn't we? We walked all around the block this afternoon. I really enjoyed myself. It was a good walk, wasn't it?"

"Yes."

"When we were looking at those beautiful flowers growing in front of our neighbor's house, we couldn't think of their names and you thought we should go the plant nursery to see if they can tell us. We can go later this week, if you like. Does that sound good?"

(*See also:* Body Language; Coaching; Communication; Crowds; Music; Walking)

SITTING AND SITTERCISES   Grandma needs exercise but she doesn't move well enough to take walks anymore. Instead, the two of you can sit in straight-back chairs facing each other and do sitting exercises. Later on you can bring these exercises to your share care group, making them even more fun when they are shared with others.

It will help your grandmother when you do these exercises with her. Do the following exercises three to five times each. Use gentle movements with a slow and deliberate pace, especially when bending

down and rising up again. Avoid jerky movements and skip an exercise if your grandmother complains about pain. If she has physical
problems, be sure to check these exercises with her doctor or physical
therapist.

> Raise your arms, breathe in. Lower your arms, exhale.

> Extend your arms in front of you, palms up, then lower
> your arms..

> Reach down the sides of your legs to touch your toes.

> Bend your chin to your chest, then look up at the
> ceiling.

> Raise your shoulders up to your ears.

> Lean forward, then pull back to row. Sing "Row, Row,
> Row Your Boat."

> Extend one arm in front of you, then move it to your
> opposite shoulder. Repeat with the other arm.

> Raise your arms, breathe in. Lower your arms, exhale.

> Stretch your arms out in front of you and scissor them.

> Stretch one leg up slowly, then stretch your other leg.

> Stretch one arm to the ceiling, then stretch the other
> arm.

> Keep your heels on the floor. Pull your toes up and
> hold for three seconds.

> Keep your toes on the floor. Pull your heels up and
> hold for three seconds.

> Raise your arms, breathe in. Lower your arms, exhale.

> Extend your arms out in front, make fists, then open
> your hands.

E

➤ Keep your arms out front and wiggle your fingers.

➤ Extend both legs in front of you, point your toes out, then flex up.

➤ Stretch your arms out front, bend your wrists down, then bend them up.

➤ Keep your arms out in front of you and make circles with your wrists.

➤ Shake out your arms.

➤ Raise one knee up toward your chest, then the other knee.

➤ Raise your arms, breathe in. Lower your arms, exhale.

➤ Put your hands on your shoulders, raise up your elbows, pull your elbows back and then together in front of your chest.

➤ Place your hands on your shoulders and twist first to one side, then the other.

➤ Clasp your hands, raise them above your head, then bring them down in front between your knees, as if you were chopping.

➤ Roll your shoulders.

➤ Raise your arms, breathe in. Lower your arms, exhale.

➤ Give yourself a big hug.

(*See also*: Body Language; Coaching; Communication; Music; Walking)

Exercise

∎∎∎∎∎∎∎∎
Eye and Sight Health

Your mother used to be an avid reader. She still likes to handle her books. She reads the opening page over and over again with obvious pleasure. Often she'll read her favorite paragraph out loud to you, each time with the exact same intonations. Even if she never gets past that first page, it's still important to her that she can see well enough to read it.

E

You'll want to take her for regular checkups with an ophthalmologist, at least once a year. She'll have a thorough eye exam that will identify problems common to the elderly. The following are the conditions the doctor will look for.

Glaucoma. This is a buildup of pressure inside of the eye. Usually occurring without any symptoms, it is easily diagnosed during the course of a routine eye examination. Untreated, glaucoma causes damage to the optic nerve, with a gradual, painless loss of vision. Eyedrops are usually effective at preventing vision loss. Advanced cases may require laser treatment or other surgery.

Age-related macular degeneration. This affects the macula, the central part of the retina, the lining of the back of the eye. As the macula begins to deteriorate, the central vision becomes blurry, affecting reading and ability to discern detail. In its advanced form, people are left with large central blind spots, seeing only in the periphery of their field of vision. Recognizing faces, watching TV, and reading become impossible.

Treatment with vitamins may be helpful in slowing down the progression in some cases. Leakage, associated with wet macular degeneration, can sometimes be treated with laser and photodynamic therapy.

Cataract. This is a term used to describe a clouding of the lens of the eye. It develops in everyone as they age, but does not always require treatment. If the vision becomes blurry as a result of a cataract, treatment involves removal of the cloudy lens and replacement with a new clear lens, called a *lens implant*. Surgery involves using ultrasound to break up and vacuum out the cloudy lens. Lasers are used to treat films that may develop years after surgery. The surgery is usually quick and is easily tolerated by the elderly, typically being done in ten minutes or less under a local anesthetic.

Diabetic retinopathy. Diabetes causes leakage from the tiny blood vessels in the back of the eye. The leakage, if untreated, causes blurring of the vision. More advanced diabetes causes fragile blood vessels to break and bleed inside the eye. This results in severe vision loss. Treatment involves the use of a laser to reduce the leakage, or more advanced surgical techniques to remove the blood from the back of the eye.

(*See also:* Alternative Remedies; Body Language; Diet and Nutrition; Health; Vitamins)

F

■ ■ ■ ■ ■ ■ ■

Family

Taking care of an Alzheimer's person ought to be a family project, although, typically, the burden falls on a single family member. If this is you, reach out to your siblings and request relief. In case you're lucky enough that they live nearby, you can expect them to share in the responsibilities, visits, and outings. It will help all of you to agree on a regular schedule. There is no way your family can empathize with you unless they can share in your experiences.

If they live out of town and your father can't travel, invite them to stay at your place where they can look after him. When they do come to your home, take advantage of the respite by actually going away somewhere. You know that if you stick around, you'll continue to be responsible for the work involved.

A few days will barely give your siblings a taste of your daily life, but on the positive side, the experience might give them a chance to bond with your father. It isn't that you're trying to prove anything to your siblings so much as you just need to make it clear to them that you need and deserve their help, support, and understanding. Taking care of your father is a family responsibility, so insist that your siblings participate in that care.

Suppose you're hosting a large family gathering, the first since the start of your father's decline. Your family is coming from out of town and they haven't seen your father in quite a while. You've called everyone before their arrival to give them a clear picture of your father's current state. You've carefully explained how to communicate with him. For example, you've told them to avoid using the phrase "Do you remember?" You've made a particularly strong point of discouraging the use of baby talk and talking about him within his earshot.

So what happens? When they arrive, your father is sweet and positively lucid, at least at certain moments. Somehow he instinctively knows to keep quiet enough to cover up his confusion. He even responds to the dreaded "Do you remember?" questions with an innocuously firm, "That sure was something!"

At this point, you suspect your siblings are probably convinced that you have grossly exaggerated your father's condition. You try to tell your brother that your father's behavior today is unusual, but you can see your brother's skepticism in his expression.

Through it all, your dad has a wonderful time, and thanks to his flawless behavior, the family is still ignorant of the challenging experiences you confront daily while caring for him. However, you can take advantage of the situation; while everyone's feeling so positive about Dad, ask your siblings to share in the caregiving in order to give you a break. Persist until you get commitments from each of them for specific dates when your father can visit them.

(*See also:* Communication; Crowds; Respite; Visitors)

■ ■ ■ ■ ■ ■ ■ ■

Fixations

There's no way of knowing why an Alzheimer's person suddenly starts fixating on one thing. When it happens, go with the flow. You probably will not be able to change the situation. If it's driving you to distraction, try a diversion that has been successful in the past. For example, suppose that all of a sudden your wife won't eat if there's more than one item on her plate, or she separates the mixed vegetables into little piles, which are cold by the time she starts to eat. After a few weeks of watching this, you can adjust your cooking and serving to suit her new habits. Serve one food item at a time during a meal.

Imagine you're out for a stroll, holding your wife by the arm, when you realize she's not looking where she's going. She's focused on fingering the buttons on her blouse. You get her attention for a minute or so, but then she's back to fussing with the buttons. She succeeds in undoing a few of them. This new behavior persists whenever she wears a blouse with buttons. The simplest solution is to change to pullover tops and back-closing tops.

Or suppose your husband manages to find the tiniest specks. He finds them, real or imaginary, on the car seat, on your friend's jacket, on the windowsill, and on his plate. He laboriously picks up these tiny specks and holds them in his fingers. If you try to convince him that he can let them go, he may get upset and insist on holding them. If you present him with a container specially labeled "Specks," he may finally relinquish them.

(*See also:* Diversions; Obsessive Behavior; Signs)

F

■ ■ ■ ■ ■ ■ ■
Foot Care

In her day, your aunt never missed her bimonthly pedicures. You've been doing your best to keep them up because they always make her feel good. Lately, however, she has been making funny little noises when she walks. Because of her dementia she may not be able to tell you what's bothering her. Her toenails could be rubbing against the front of her shoe, making every step uncomfortable, or perhaps her shoes don't fit properly anymore. Also she might have bunions, corns, or calluses that are too subtle for you to detect. Look for reddish areas and feel her skin. Calluses may not be visible but they can be warm to the touch. If left untreated, calluses can become ulcerated or infected.

You will want to start taking your aunt to a podiatrist to have her nails clipped and her feet checked every three months. It may not be as fancy as her pedicurist, but a podiatrist can identify problems and advise you on regular care, including what would be the best footwear for her to wear. You can make up for the loss of the luxurious pedicures by giving your aunt footbaths and rubbing her feet with fragrant lotions.

Athlete's foot is another common condition that flourishes in the damp environment of socks and shoes. Walking shoes made with a "breathable" fabric provide a good way to minimize this problem.

If your aunt is a diabetic, you'll want to be extra vigilant and talk to her podiatrist about the additional care you may need to give her at home.

(*See also:* Body Language; Health)

■ ■ ■ ■ ■ ■ ■
F Forgetfulness

See: Alzheimer's Disease; Coaching; Choices; Comunication; Dementia; Visitors; Word Substitutions

■ ■ ■ ■ ■ ■ ■
Forgiveness

Often, matters will come up in your caregiving experiences that will certainly enrage you and bring out feelings that have been buried for ages. You're apt to become very angry and frustrated. So, forgiveness is very important when you're dealing with such intensely emotional and stressful situations; but often this is easier said than done. Start by forgiving yourself for your feelings, and acknowledge that they come with the territory.

For example, your sister has been a thorn in your side for a long time now. Ever since your mother came to live with you, your sister has criticized your every decision and action. She won't come to see for herself what's going on, but in her mind there's nothing you can do right. You're fed up with the hostility she evokes in you. When the phone rings on Saturday mornings, you get a sinking feeling in your stomach and the anger rises in your throat as you realize it's your sister's weekly telephone call.

So far you've had sole responsibility for your mother, so you know you don't have to put up with this kind of harassment. Yet you feel guilty about your negative reactions because, after all, she is your sister and you're supposed to love each other. You've tried to tell her that her attitude hurts you, but she doesn't seem to listen. She makes you angry and unhappy, so now it's time for you to take a stand and tell her that you don't want any more negative phone calls. Write a note to your sister and let her know your new resolution: positive phone calls or no telephone calls at all. Insist that she take her turn caring for your mother and perhaps she'll realize that her judgments of you have been too harsh.

When you are confronted with angry, hostile feelings, give yourself ten or fifteen minutes to acknowledge your anger, wallow in it, and then let it go, while you forgive yourself for just being human. If these feelings continue to bother you, talk to your counselor or therapist.

F

Suppose some things took place between you and your father when you were a kid that still trigger unresolved anger and hurt in you. Now your father is living with you because he has dementia, but he has absolutely no recollection of those events from so long ago. As much as you try to stifle it, the rage still sometimes wells up inside you and it makes living with your father very difficult. You've heard about the importance of forgiveness, but your father's dementia makes it impossible to talk to him about past events.

Forgiving him without a confrontation and acknowledgment on his part is virtually impossible for you. How can you deal with old wrongs when the perpetrator has grown old and demented? Confronting him with the truth at this point may give you some relief, although it might disturb your father so much that he will retreat even further and become either deeply depressed or overtly angry and agitated, which will make your life with him even more difficult. Is it worth it? You might decide that your father is a different person now and try to accept him as he is. You may be able to forgive yourself for feeling anger or rage at the man you used to know.

There are times when outrage is appropriate, as in the case of physical abuse, molestation, and violence. If you recognize that your feelings about what happened are real, and what your father did was unforgivable, your rage is justified. With the help of a counselor you may be able to make peace in your heart with your past, even if your father doesn't acknowledge any of it. You need to find release from this pain and you deserve to be set free in order to grow and move on.

(*See also:* Counseling; Family; Guilt; Support Groups)

■ ■ ■ ■ ■ ■ ■
Friends

F

Your husband, who has Alzheimer's, is fortunate enough to have an old friend living nearby. The old friend also has Alzheimer's. You've made arrangements with the friend's caregiver so they can spend time together at least once a month. Your husband's friend is about as confused as your husband is, but the two of them still have such a good time when they get together to reminisce about old times.

By now, you're quite used to hearing the same old stories repeated again and again whenever the two of them get together, and you've come to realize that their stories aren't important; they're just a way to express the love they share for each other. As you sit back and watch, you see them as they are to each other: a couple of high school kids. This is a priceless time for both of them and you feel privileged to be able to share it. If you have access to a video camera or a tape recorder, this would be a good time to use it.

We all need friends and people we can relate to, no matter what our mental state is. You're doing an amazing job as a caregiver, but as much as you try, you cannot provide the kind of companionship that a friend can give.

Your grandma came to live with you from her home in another state. You realize that she needs friends of her own, but her social skills are pretty much gone, so she relies on you for her total companionship. Your share care group's been good for her, because she's become friends with one of the women. Neither of them remembers the other's name, but that doesn't seem to matter. The two of them greet each other as long-lost friends whenever they meet. You and the other caregivers help them out with their conversations; otherwise they'd probably remain silent throughout the whole visit. During lulls in the conversation, you may be uncomfortable with the silence, but notice that they seem totally content just being there with each other.

(*See also:* Communication; Conversations; Share Care)

■ ■ ■ ■ ■ ■ ■ ■

Future

Making plans is synonymous with "the future." We all need to feel we have some sort of future, although, in reality, we know nothing is ever a certainty for any of us. "Planning" what you'd like to do in the future can be a cheerful experience. Just think about the times you've fantasized about winning the lottery!

Your father is big on making plans. When you were a kid, the family's summer vacation was already planned long before the daffodils even began to bloom. Now your dad relishes discussing the next day's doings, which may be real or fanciful, because by morning he may have forgotten most of them. Should he remember something that doesn't fit in with your plans, you can redirect him with an enthusiastic alternative; for example, say something like, "I have a surprise for you. The other day you wanted to go to the library (or the store) but it was closed. Well, we can go today. How about that? That's good news, isn't it?"

Your father has wonderful memories of family picnics when he was a child. All through your childhood you'd hear stories about these legendary events, although he can't really talk about them lucidly anymore. Now, whenever you want him to feel really special, suggest planning a picnic just like the old days, "You know, it's supposed to be beautiful weather on Sunday. That's what the weather reporter said on the news. How about a picnic in the park? We could go to the deli and get a picnic lunch like your mother used to make."

You can spend a whole evening planning your picnic (real or not), right down to the very last detail. Food is one of the best topics for daydreaming together, and in the process you can recall one of his favorite childhood memories.

"You know, Dad, I've been thinking we should take a visit to that little hideaway you like so much. There's that neat bookstore and café where we can read some good books and eat lunch. They make great turkey sandwiches with avocados and sprouts. Then later we'll drive around the corner to the ice cream parlor and have a big scoop of ice cream in a sugar cone. What flavor would you like? Chocolate with almonds? Kiwi fruit with macadamia nuts? Or Guinness stout ice cream with beer nuts?"

F

Make it up as you go along, making sure to include your father's favorite foods. His responses will tell you where to go next. The point is that you're not making a promise; you're merely painting possibilities for the future.

(*See also*: Empathy; Reality; Validation)

F

G

■ ■ ■ ■ ■ ■ ■ ■

Games

We're never too old to play games and we all have our favorites, whether bingo, bridge, canasta, jacks, tiddlywinks, horseshoes, ring toss, badminton, Ping-Pong, or pin the tail on the donkey.

Mental stimulation continues to be extremely important for your mother. If she enjoys crossword puzzles and other word games, look for game books in the magazine section of your supermarket. You'll find books for varying abilities, so you can select the appropriate level. Your mother needs to be challenged but not overwhelmed. When she reaches a point when even simple crossword puzzles and other word games are too difficult for her to do on her own, she can "help" you instead.

CARD GAMES   Your husband may not be able to play card games anymore, but you can create simplified, noncompetitive versions of the ones that he used to enjoy. Perhaps he used to like playing bridge, so you can make up a new "game" vaguely reminiscent of bridge. Start by dealing each of you a few cards and then take turns laying down the cards according to suits. The purpose of the game can be to see how quickly you both can lay them out. Your husband also may be able to play a game of solitaire, as long as you play it with him.

He might be able to play open-handed poker. You do that by drawing five cards from the pile and laying them face up on the table. Together you can decide which cards to keep and which ones to discard or replace. You can keep going until you have a decent poker hand, no matter how long it takes to get a good one.

There's nothing wrong with games of competition as long as your husband has fun playing them. If you notice that he's becoming frustrated or agitated, change to a noncompetitive, nonskilled game, or simply take a break and do something else for a while.

OUTDOOR GAMES Outdoor games can be anything from tossing the ball to croquet. Beach balls are easy to toss and they are soft and gentle to catch. Go to a local toy store and buy a variety of balls in different sizes (preferably Nerf foam balls). Many children's lawn games won't feel too juvenile as long as you take them seriously. Consider ring toss, horseshoes, or lawn bowling. For safety reasons, be sure to shop for the plastic versions of these games.

(*See also*: Activities; Exercise; Personal Space; Projects; Word Games)

G

■ ■ ■ ■ ■ ■ ■ ■

Gardening

Gardening can be a relaxing and rewarding experience for a person with dementia, as long as that person is so inclined. She may have physical limitations now that you can accommodate with low stools for her to sit on for weeding and working with the soil. If she's in a wheelchair, you can set flower boxes up high enough for easy access.

Your childhood home was surrounded by vegetable gardens, herb patches, and flower beds, all tended lovingly by your mother. She's living with you now. You take her on outings, you cook together, and once in a while you get a chance to read with her, but there are long periods of time when you're distracted with your own work and your mother is left to her own devices.

She goes out of her way not to disturb you when you're working and spends most of her time wandering around the house. You've tried to set up an "office" for her but she's not interested, so you don't know what else you can do. Then one morning you ask her where she'd like to go for the day's outing and she says, "The nursery; it's time for spring planting." Aha! You had forgotten about her old passion for horticulture.

Start with a single flower box. Encourage your mother as she selects seeds, plant food, gloves, potting soil, trowel, and watering can. Before long she will be tending two more flower boxes, which makes getting around the apartment a bit tricky, but the maneuvering is worth it just to see the joy on your mother's face when the first green shoots appear.

If you're lucky enough to have a yard, you can set up a small area for your mother to plant a vegetable or flower garden. You'll probably have to pitch in and help her, but later you can enjoy the fruits of your labors with a special dinner of homegrown vegetables. A bouquet of flowers grown in the garden would also be very nice.

(*See also:* Activities; Kitchen; Outings; Personal Space; Projects; Validation)

G

■ ■ ■ ■ ■ ■ ■ ■
Going Home

A person with Alzheimer's loses most of her current memory or it becomes so fractured that it doesn't make any sense to her. Your aunt may have lived with you for years, but your home may still feel strange to her at those times when she regresses into an altered reality. Since most of her intact memories are now centered in her childhood, she has a strong urge to return to that familiar place.

Wanting to "go home" is common among Alzheimer's people. When this happens, the kindest thing you can do for your aunt is to acknowledge her desire, but then provide her with a reasonable distraction. There may be times when a simple distraction doesn't work, and then you may have to ease her mind by telling her a "loving lie."

Every so often your sister will stand at the front door with a load of clothes in her arms and with great determination she will announce: "I'm going home! I have to leave now. Just leave me alone! I don't want any favors from anybody. I don't want any rides or anything like that. So, I'm going to walk and it's twenty miles, so I have to leave right now!"

In the past you've tried reasoning with her, reminding her that she sold her condo and moved across the country to live with you, but when you do this she gets very angry and accuses you of lying to her and keeping her a prisoner.

Sometimes she'll announce: "I have to go home now. My mother's waiting for me and she'll get very angry if I'm not on time." At that point it becomes clear to you that there's something else going on. It's not simply a matter of returning to her own condo; she's talking about her childhood. Put your arm around her and say, "Mother called and she'll come over here later. But she insisted we should go ahead and eat dinner now."

On the other hand, your sister may still be aware on some level that your mother is no longer alive. In that case, be very gentle with her as you explain, "Sis, Mother has been gone for several years now but it's still so hard for me to believe. She would always come over for dinner on Thursdays, and even after all these years there are times when I find myself setting that extra place for her . . . But I'm so glad that you're living here with me now."

This kind of scene could be an indication that your sister is feeling insecure, lonely, or without purpose. Getting her involved in fixing up her personal space would be good diversion.

Or you can start a project that the two of you will enjoy doing together. It could be something that she used to enjoy, such as sewing, gardening, or cooking. You could say, "Before you go, Sis, would you please help me with the salad dressing. I love that special recipe of yours and I just don't have the hang of it yet." You don't want to argue with her about her wanting to leave, but simply suggest a postponement. With a good distraction, she will soon have forgotten about her original intentions.

Your diversion should be a project that's short and manageable in order to give your sister a sense of accomplishment. She may be painfully slow now, stretching your patience since you wind up doing most of the work, but you'll succeed in making her feel useful and involved. When the project is finished, give her a good hug and a sincere compliment. "I'm sure glad you're helping me with this. It would have taken me forever to do this without you. Thank you so much."

(See also: Affection; Compliments; Diversions; Loving Lies; Personal Space; Reality)

Going Home

■ ■ ■ ■ ■ ■ ■ ■

Guilt

Your brother's not able to respond to you with positive reactions any-more, so the assurance you might need to let you know that you're doing the right thing may be replaced by doubt and guilt.

You're doing so well with your brother that your friends have nominated you for sainthood. Most of the time this is great to hear, but there are other times when heavy feelings of guilt envelop you because you feel that you could do so much more. Your relationship with your brother has become more and more lopsided as you con-stantly give, while he constantly takes. You're aware that the circum-stances make this inevitable, but as your situation becomes more extreme, you may find yourself questioning your own feelings and actions. We're all used to getting strokes or feedback from the people affected by our good deeds.

You cannot help but feel burdened with this task you've taken on, and you may find yourself envious and resentful of your siblings or friends who are free to pursue their own lives. If you're trying to jug-gle your brother's caregiving with a full-time job while taking care of your own family, then you definitely have a full plate. You may get a lot of help from your family but still feel it's your responsibility, and there may be times when you are overwhelmed with guilt for inevita-bly neglecting one or the other.

When you blame your brother, you are only being human in blaming his condition for your situation. There may even be times when you wish he would die so it would all be over. It's very hard for us to talk about these "dark" thoughts or to even admit to ourselves that we harbor them. However, we've all felt them at one time or another, so forgive yourself for being normal.

The next time your brother drives you to the edge, take a deep breath and find a diversion for him so you can retreat to the most peaceful place in your house and have a good cry. Or give yourself a good hug and promise yourself to take some real time off in the very near future. Tomorrow night get a sitter for your brother and go to a movie or dinner with friends. Look into respite care that will give you some time for yourself on a more regular basis.

G

As your brother's condition deteriorates, you know that it's only a matter of time before you'll no longer be able to care for him at home. You've started looking into care facilities in your area, but you have a heavy heart because you feel the weight of guilt and a sense of failure. You know that it's important for your brother to have what's best for him, and as hard as it may be to admit this, that might ultimately be a care facility. Your rational self knows there is no reason for you to feel guilty. After all, you've given him a home for a long time now, and you know that even if he moves into a care facility, you will still be there for him.

Your feelings and thoughts are normal. Try to share them with your Alzheimer's Association support group, even if it is very hard to talk about them. Start by discussing the weakest negative feelings and then work your way up to the really frightening ones. Everyone in the group will most likely share your feelings of guilt over very similar issues. If this subject has not yet been dealt with, the group will probably be relieved that it has finally been broached. You are involved in a tremendous undertaking, so you're entitled to dark thoughts and doubts like any other normal human being. Our culture disapproves of negative thinking and we've been scolded since childhood for expressing negative thoughts, so when they pop up, they automatically trigger our guilt reflexes.

If you feel overwhelmed and these feelings are so frequent that they interfere with your personal well-being and your effectiveness as a caregiver, then talk to your family about one of them taking over the caregiving for a while. At the very least, insist that a family member stay at your house for a couple of weeks or longer so you can take a vacation.

You may feel selfish to want time for yourself and this can lead to additional guilt feelings. However, needing a break doesn't mean that you're letting your brother down or that you've failed. A much-needed break gives you a chance to think about your situation and realize that you've undertaken the most difficult task of your life and that, on the whole, you're doing a fine job.

(*See also:* Care Facilities; Counseling; Family; Forgiveness; Respite; Support Groups)

H

■ ■ ■ ■ ■ ■ ■ ■
Hallucinations

Your friend Alicia's hallucinations are totally real to her. To help her come back to reality, you can "go into the space" with her to help her remedy the situation, and then you'll be able to divert her. "Going into the space" with her means that you will join her in her experience, with empathy and sensitivity. When you are able to feel what she's feeling, you're more likely to be successful in bringing her back to the present.

Suppose one day you're having lunch with Alicia, when she suddenly exclaims, "Get that bear out of here!" You may start to protest that there's nothing there, but you stop yourself. Take a deep breath as you get up and say to her, "I bet he's one hungry bear. I'll take him outside and feed him."

Go through the motions of taking the "bear" out of the room, closing the door behind you. When you return, use a serious tone when you say, "It's a good thing you told me. He was really hungry, so I gave him something to eat and now he's gone back to the woods. Are you ready for some more iced tea?"

(*See also:* Diversions; Empathy; Honesty; Loving Lies; Reality; Validation)

■ ■ ■ ■ ■ ■ ■ ■
Health

Older people are generally more susceptible to infections, adverse drug reactions, and other health problems. Nutrition, exercise, and regular physical checkups are very important. Hopefully, you can find a doctor who has had some experience with the elderly. It's also a good idea to establish a relationship with the doctor's support staff. You can call them for general advice, and with their guidance you can often solve problems that may not be serious enough to require a visit to the doctor's office.

GENERAL CHECKUPS

As far as you can tell, your mother is doing well, but you're extra vigilant about her health because she can no longer tell you when she's not feeling well. You make sure she eats a healthy diet and take her for a physical checkup on a regular basis. Before you take your mother for her physical, you will want to do some homework. Make a list of her intake of food and liquids and bring all her medications and supplements with you to the doctor's office. Write down your specific concerns. It is easier to think of details when you are free of pressure. You can give everything to the nurse as you sign in, to give the doctor a chance to review the materials ahead of time.

On your first visit to a new doctor, you will want to discuss communication. Let the staff know that you're concerned that your mother should be part of the conversation or discussion, even if her lack of verbal skill makes it hard for her to participate fully. Most doctors who deal with the memory-impaired on a regular basis will acknowledge the Alzheimer's patient while still getting the important information from you. If your mother's doctor ignores her or treats her like a child, speak up and let him know that she will likely understand what is being said about her, even if she can't respond, and that she doesn't appreciate being talked to as if she were a baby.

When you arrive at the doctor's office, calmly explain to your mother why she's there. Say, "Mom, we're here for your checkup. We do this every six months. You seem to be doing just fine; we're just making double sure that everything is still working well. First we're going to go into the nurse's office, so she can check your vital signs. She's going to take your blood pressure and your temperature and stuff like that."

When it's necessary, say, "The nurse is going to weigh you now. We'll both help you get up on the scale. Okay? We won't let you fall, you hear?" So there you are in the exam room, waiting, and, of course, within minutes your mother asks again where you are and what you're doing there. So you start all over again. "We're here for your checkup; there's nothing wrong, as far as we know, and now we're going to be in here and wait for the doctor to take a look at you. Is there anything you'd like to talk to the doctor about?"

When you ask her for her input, that will give her a feeling of self-control in a situation that can be frightening. As usual, you will assume that she understands most conversations, even if she is not able to express herself.

Keep the doctor informed about any visits you have had with other health-care professionals, such as a dentist, eye doctor, or podiatrist. You may also want to have regular visits with a psychiatrist or a neurologist. It's especially important to discuss any sudden changes in your mother's health, alertness, or orientation. When she's seen these specialists, let her doctor know about any changes in her medications or treatment plans.

Be sure to ask questions. If the doctor uses terms that are unfamiliar to you, ask for an explanation. There are no questions too small or silly for a good doctor to deal with.

COMMON HEALTH CONDITIONS
There are several conditions for you to be aware of and discuss with your mother's doctor: Ask for a description of symptoms and recommendations on actions you should take if these symptoms develop. Some of these conditions may be harmless and a trip to the emergency room could cause further trauma and might in fact be useless.

> **TIA (transient ischaemic attack) ministrokes.** The Alzheimer's person may momentarily lose movement of the right or left side of the body, or speech may be affected. Occasionally there may be a loss of consciousness. Call the doctor immediately and describe the event (Johnston et al. 2000). If the doctor believes a TIA occurred and the person is not already taking aspirin, you may want to discuss adding a baby aspirin once a day.
>
> Make the Alzheimer's person comfortable and don't be surprised if there's extra confusion for a while. The person will likely regain composure after a few hours. TIAs

rarely leave any detectable symptoms. If any remain, it is a sign of a slightly more serious stroke, but even these can slowly improve over days to weeks.

Vagal response. The vagus nerve controls certain automatic functions in the body, for instance, helping to regulate heartbeat and acid secretions in the stomach. A vagal response can be caused by stress, overheating, or a sudden increase in digestive activity. It often happens right after a heavy or rich meal and is very frightening when it happens. The person may throw up and pass out. A vagal response usually isn't life threatening.

H

You'll want to lay the person down flat, preferably on his or her side to ease breathing and give him or her time to regain composure. You may see some drowsiness for a several hours afterward. The doctor should be informed any time there's a loss of consciousness, because sometimes the cause is not that clear and it could be either a treatable condition or a serious one, like heart arrhythmia (Horton 2002).

Osteoporosis. Many elderly individuals have weakened bones. Alzheimer's people are especially prone to falls, which are the most common cause of fractures, usually of the hip or the wrist. However, they can also fracture ribs or vertebrae easily. Even a deep sneeze or a firm grip can cause a bone to break.

Since they tend to wander, Alzheimer's people are particularly prone to falls, especially after their condition has progressed to the point of including the impairment of motor skills as simple as walking. To help avoid falls, consider removing small throw rugs, low stools, or ottomans. Also consider installing handrails in bathtubs and at the toilet. A commode at the bedside can lessen the likelihood of an unsupervised trip to the bathroom with its attendant risk of a bad fall.

Senile purpura. This is a purple discoloration of the skin, which usually occurs on the limbs, especially the forearms and shins. It can be caused by a simple firm grip. Caused by leaks from tiny blood vessels under the skin, it may or may not go away by itself. Younger people have layers of fat, which disguise this kind of common bruising. It can often look like a serious bruise and may appear ominous to outsiders, who may mistake it for signs of physical abuse (Feinstein et al. 1973).

Skin tears. As we age we, lose the protective fat layer in our skin and it can become very fragile. Lather your mother's body in rich lotions as much as possible. Some of her skin may be so fragile that large tears can occur. They may look serious, but they usually heal without needing stitches. However, they do need to be carefully bandaged. Some special dressings are available for this problem. Call your doctor for advice and guidance.

H

Urinary tract infections (UTIs). UTIs are common in the elderly. Older men often have prostate enlargement, which predisposes them to UTIs. In both men and women, urination becomes painful with a burning sensation and there's an urge to urinate frequently. You also may notice that the urine is darker than normal and has an unusually strong scent. You should consult your doctor, who will likely prescribe antibiotics. Cranberry juice is often recommended. Note that dehydration is one common cause of UTIs.

An unrecognized UTI, or for that matter any infection, can cause a sudden dramatic worsening of confusion and all the other symptoms of Alzheimer's. When the condition is treated, the Alzheimer's person often will improve. That's why it's so important to see a doctor for any sudden changes in the mental state of the patient.

(*See also:* Alternative Remedies; Alzheimer's Disease; Alzheimer's Medications; Appetite; Death and Dying; Dementia; Dental Health; Diet and Nutrition; Exercise; Eye and Sight Health; Foot Care; Hospital; Incontinence; Medication; Paperwork; Pills; Stress; Vitamins)

■ ■ ■ ■ ■ ■ ■ ■
Hearing Health

Your mother appears to have problems with her hearing lately. You may be wondering if you need to get her a hearing aid. You take her to a hearing center for tests and discover that it's only a serious accumulation of wax in her ears. A quick cleaning will take care of the problem. After this visit, you decide to take her back for regular visits every few months.

If it turns out that your mother is, in fact, hard of hearing, you have some tough decisions to make. People have to learn how to use a hearing aid, which may be virtually impossible for an Alzheimer's person. Even when an Alzheimer's person has used a hearing aid before, she may have difficulties with the adjustments.

If your mother is hard of hearing, there are some remedies available over the counter. For television viewing, you can get a cordless set of headphones, and for general use you can get Mom a sound amplifier, which works with a simple earplug. With the latter, just be aware that Mom's own speech will be amplified as well, which is likely to startle her.

(*See also:* Body Language; Health)

■ ■ ■ ■ ■ ■ ■ ■
Hoarding

Hiding and hoarding are common among Alzheimer's people. Usually it's harmless, but you'll want to check drawers frequently, in case the hidden objects are food items that can spoil and not only stink, but also become a health hazard. Wastebaskets, pockets, and shoes are other favorite hiding places, especially for glasses, dentures, and hearing aids.

Suppose one day while you are cleaning your sister's room, you find two bars of soap stashed under her bed. Several days later, you discover two more bars in the top drawer of her bureau. No wonder you're running out of soap in the bathroom! You explain to your sister that the soap is supposed to be kept in the bathroom and she nods impatiently because, of course, she knows that bar soap belongs in the bathroom. But it's likely that she'll forget what you've just told her ten minutes from now.

Your sister is a child of the Depression and has always been a fanatic about saving things, even tiny slivers of soap, so you decide to try a different approach. Get a basket, put a sign on it saying "Soap" and put it on top of her chest of drawers. Fill it with the slivers of soap from her various hiding places. After a few weeks, you can suggest that she keep the basket of soap in the bathroom instead. Buy liquid soap for use in the bathroom, since you know she doesn't understand how to use it, and she will be likely to leave it alone.

If this doesn't work, or if she's hoarding a variety of different items, consider installing childproof locks on all the cabinets and drawers so you can lock up anything that you don't want your sister to hoard. Continue checking her room frequently for stashes, but it wouldn't hurt to leave a few of her favorites in place.

(*See also:* Home Safety; Signs)

H

■ ■ ■ ■ ■ ■ ■ ■

Home Help

You've decided you need help looking after your father. Until now, you've been doing everything by yourself: all the cleaning, cooking, and caring for yourself and your father. Your energy is depleted by the routine maintenance, leaving you with little time or energy for any pleasure or stimulation for the two of you. Here are some possible options on home help.

FAMILY   Your first conversation should be with your siblings and other family members. If they live out of town, ask them to come and stay with your father for several days or a week at a time. If your father can still travel, have him stay at their homes for a change. Be very insistent with them; this is the kind of situation where everyone must pitch in. Caring for your father should be a responsibility that is shared by all of you.

If they live nearby, you can work out a regular schedule to give yourself respite at least one day a week. At the very least, ask them to help every so often by cleaning your house or cooking a meal. This will free you up to do something more enjoyable with your father.

HOUSEKEEPER

If you can afford to, you can hire a full-time housekeeper to help with daily household chores and upkeep, or you could consider hiring a part-time person to come in once or twice a week to do the laundry and the floors. It's very likely this person will interact with your dad, so make sure that you share some of this book to help the person in communicating with your father.

PERSONAL CARE AIDE

If your dad has problems with physically getting around, you can hire a personal care aide to come in daily or even just a few times a week to help him with his baths, shaving, or any other physical situations that you may need assistance with. You can check with your local agency on aging for referrals to qualified agencies or individuals. Be sure that anytime you consider hiring a private aide, you check references and qualifications.

PERSONAL COMPANION

If you're working full-time and there is no access to adult day care, you might consider hiring a companion for him. This person can provide your father with intellectual stimulation by spending time with him in your home, and by reading, conversing, or playing games with him. A companion can take your dad out on picnics, to the library or museum, and to other places he might enjoy. You might want to check with a nearby college to see if there are any students interested in a job.

It's important, of course, that Dad enjoys the company of his companion and that they're compatible. Besides checking applicants' references, you'll want to make sure they are open to new ideas and approaches in caring for a person with Alzheimer's. While your potential assistant interacts with Dad, observe them. Does he treat your father respectfully? Do they seem to enjoy each other's company? Your father's new companion should have a few trial runs (under your supervision) using the approaches outlined in this book so that he will understand how you expect your father to be treated.

(*See also:* Day Care; Family; Respite; Share Care; Support Groups)

■ ■ ■ ■ ■ ■ ■ ■
Home Safety

There are several safety measures you can take without having to remodel your entire house. It's worth hiring a professional to install safety bars, shutoff valves for the water, and concealed switches for electrical hazards. The kitchen and bathroom are primary trouble spots, but don't forget about garages and storage sheds.

WINDOWS AND DOORS Your front door should have a lock that your mother cannot open by herself, something like a double dead bolt. Also, place a stop sign or a sign on the door that reads, "Do not go out this door." You can position similar signs on any other doors that you want to keep secure. If that fails to work, try hanging a curtain in front of the door or installing a full-length mirror on the door.

If you live in an upper-level apartment, make sure that all your windows are secured and have appropriate screens. If you have a balcony, secure the door; but go ahead and use the balcony with your mother whenever the weather permits.

If you are in a rural area and your mother is prone to wandering, you'll need to have your yard securely fenced with locks on the gates and make sure that she always wears an identification bracelet.

KITCHEN If your mother likes to fiddle around in the kitchen but you're worried about accidents, you can take precautions by making a few safety changes.

Kitchen checklist:

- ‣ Keep sharp knives out of reach.

- ‣ Use childproof closures for any cabinets that you want to secure.

- ‣ Keep all household cleaning stuff out of reach.

- ‣ Keep small appliances unplugged or off the counters.

- ‣ Remove the knobs from the stove.

- ‣ Remove the stopper from the sink.

- ‣ Unplug the garbage disposal and dishwasher.

BATHROOM   You will want to install grab bars in the tub or shower and place a large safety mat in the tub or shower if it doesn't already have a nonskid bottom. You can either install a grab bar by the toilet or use a free-standing safety rail.

If your father routinely turns on the water and leaves it running, you can avoid flooding by removing the stoppers in all your sinks and tubs and installing a water shutoff ball valve under the sink. As an added safety measure, turn your water heater's thermostat down to a tolerable temperature to keep him from scalding himself.

Bath times will be much easier and less contentious if you use a hand-held shower in place of the stationary showerhead. When you first turn it on and lead Dad into the shower, let the showerhead hang down. It's less frightening that way.

Transfer all medication out of the medicine cabinet and into a cabinet that's inaccessible to your father. You will also want to keep all household cleaning solutions out of reach. It's too easy for your father to confuse mouthwash with dishwashing liquid, especially if they both have a lemony smell.

FIRE SAFETY Review your house for anything that can cause accidents. Your aunt means well, but she doesn't always remember what she's been doing. She may have turned on the stove with the intention of making you a cup of coffee, and then forgotten all about it. If matches and lighters represent a temptation to her, you will want to keep them out of her reach. It's lovely to have dinner by candlelight, but make sure you don't leave the lit candles unattended. Buy a couple of fire extinguishers and place them in strategic spots, like the kitchen and near the living room. Have them inspected annually by the fire department.

(*See also:* Identification; Neighborhood Flyer; Safe Return; Signs; Wandering)

H

■ ■ ■ ■ ■ ■ ■ ■

Honesty

Most of us have had truth telling pounded into our heads from early childhood. However, as a caregiver, you will often find yourself faced with the altered reality that occurs with Alzheimer's. As an Alzheimer's person regresses into the past and loses touch with the present, you will find that you'll be more successful by going into the past with the person. This will often mean that you'll have to resort to what sounds like a lie to you, but it is, in fact, the Alzheimer's person's truth because it's based upon his or her reality.

Your father is still cognizant of many events in his life and you're usually able to discuss them honestly with him whenever he brings them up. Your mother died quite a few years ago and Dad remembers that fact most of the time. Yet there are other times when he slips into a long-ago reality as he anxiously waits for her to come home. Most of the time you should be able to help him recall that she has died, but there may be other times when he will become agitated and accuse you of lying to him.

At those times when he cannot hear the truth, you may have to resort to telling him a loving lie, even though your family has always been sticklers for honesty. It may feel awkward at first, but you will realize that there are some moments when a slight untruth is the kindest response you can give to him. In order to be convincing, however, your loving lies should be realistic and based on a truth of some kind. For example, you might say, "Mom will be late. She wants us to go ahead and eat our dinner now. She didn't say what time she'll be here."

If your mother was an intellectual, then use an answer that would have fit in with her real interests. You could say something like, "She had to stop at the library to do some research. She was always so serious about her research, wasn't she? How about the two of us going to the library tomorrow? Or maybe the hardware store. What do you think?"

In this way you will gently turn the conversation away from his concern about your mother and channel it into something involving your relationship with him.

Suppose your wife has been diagnosed with Alzheimer's disease. You wonder if you should tell her the truth about the diagnosis. This is a very tough decision. If she's already forgotten about the tests and the doctor's visit, then you'll probably just want to leave it alone for the time being. Nothing will change drastically in the near future, so try to relax and carry on with your lives as usual.

If your wife is still in the early stages of the disease and insists on knowing, then you'll just have to trust your instincts about what you tell her. Be aware that hearing she has Alzheimer's disease may be devastating for her. On the other hand, it can help her under-stand what's been happening to her lately. Keep in mind that science is not yet able to distinguish with certainty between different types of dementia and Alzheimer's disease. Discuss this with her, but follow up with reassurances that you'll be there for her and help her along the way.

You could say something like, "Sweetie, when we went to see the doctor today, she said you have dementia and it may be Alzhei-mer's. That means that you forget things and sometimes you get con-fused. Well, you could have told her that, right?" Then, give her a hug and continue with, "I'm so glad you're living here with me so I can help you with the remembering. And I'll always be here for you, don't you forget that!" Then change to another unrelated and more upbeat topic.

Honesty

(*See also:* Attitude; Empathy; Guilt; Loving Lies; Reality; Validation)

■ ■ ■ ■ ■ ■ ■ ■
Hospital

Hospital stays and even brief visits to the emergency room are extraordinarily traumatic for an Alzheimer's person. All too often the hospital personnel are not properly equipped or don't have the time to handle a person with dementia. Be prepared to spend a lot of time at the bedside and become involved in the care.

INPATIENT Suppose your mother has to spend time in the hospital. You would have already made sure that the word "Alzheimer's" is clearly written on the front of her chart. She fell asleep last night without any trouble and you finally went home to get some rest yourself. But you arrived this morning to find your mother wide- eyed and on the verge of tears. She was struggling against restraints tied to her wrists and ankles. You felt dizzy with anguish for her and ran to the nurses station. What had happened to cause so drastic a measure? The head nurse, in a soothing (i.e., patronizing) voice explained, "Your mother was quite unmanageable this morning. She refused to eat her breakfast and she screamed and struck out at the nurse who came to bathe her. We routinely restrain and sedate our Alzheimer's patients for their own safety. Everything will be fine. Don't worry. She doesn't understand anyway."

At this point, your guts are churning and boiling. This is your sweet mother trussed up like a Thanksgiving turkey. You know how reasonable your mother is in spite of her dementia. Didn't anyone even try to communicate with her? You may be seething as you respond to the supercilious nurse. Take not one, but two very deep breaths as you say, "I will see to it that someone is here all day with my mother. While we're here, your staff can bathe her and take care of other activities that may cause a problem. Let's do this without using any restraints or sedatives."

H

You can run a crash course for the staff on how to communicate with your mother and how to gain her confidence. Sharing this book may help. You will want to stop anyone in their tracks if they start using baby talk. If your mother has to undergo a medical procedure, ask the technician to explain it to her step-by-step, in a normal tone of voice, and repeat the details as often as necessary. If she resists bathing in these unfamiliar surroundings, ask the staff to let you help with her baths until she feels safe with them.

Hang a few of her favorite pictures on the wall that faces her bed. If there is no music or radio available, bring a small tape player from home and play the music she loves. If she's not on a restricted diet, you can supplement the hospital menu with goodies from home. You'll want to stay with her as much as you can for the next few days, so arm yourself with a substantial collection of books, pictures, puzzles, and songs. Your intention should be to have as much fun as possible, no matter how serious her condition might be.

Laughter is an amazing healing tool. Encourage her to participate as much as her physical condition will allow. Sing together and "dance" with your hands and arms to Mozart, Duke Ellington, or Aretha Franklin. This is guaranteed to look weird to anybody who peeks into her hospital room. That idea alone can provide the two of you with some good laughs. "Those other people must think we are nuts, huh? Boy, they don't know how much fun they're missing, do they? I think we should invite them to join us, don't you?"

Whatever your mother's ailment is, you want to get her back home as fast as possible. Suppose she has a broken hip: After surgery and a few days of observation in the hospital, she would normally be sent to a rehabilitation center for several weeks of physical therapy. Let her doctor know that you want to bring her home as soon as possible. Find out whether or not Medicare or Medicaid will pay for a physical therapist to come to your home.

Many hospitals have case managers who will work with you on "after care." They can help you organize a home-care solution and help you meet with social workers or occupational therapists in order to retrofit your home to suit your mother's special needs if necessary.

OUTPATIENT Your grandfather has to go to the hospital as an outpatient. To keep him from becoming unnecessarily anxious, wait until you're on the way to the hospital before you explain to him what's going to happen. He'll take his cues from your attitude and words. Stay calm and upbeat, but be straightforward and honest about what to expect, and then reassure him that you'll be there with him.

The hospital usually requires patients to arrive a couple of hours ahead of time. You know that your grandfather would go nuts waiting that long, so you call the supervisor and tell her that he has Alzheimer's, so you need to know the absolute latest possible arrival time. Also ask her to double-check to make sure that "Alzheimer's" is written big and bold on the cover of your grandfather's chart. Amazingly, hospital personnel are often not prepared to handle special situations like dementia and Alzheimer's.

H

Stay with your grandfather through all the prepping, explaining the procedures to him, perhaps not correctly, but at least convincingly. If he is going to have only a local anesthesia, you can stay with him throughout the procedure to help him remain calm. Explain everything as it's happening and remind him why he's there in the first place. Say something like, "Grandaddy, we're at the hospital to have a cataract removed from your right eye. You'll be able to see so much better afterward. Isn't that great? Right now the nurse is going to give you some eyedrops to help numb your eye, okay? I'll be right here with you."

If your grandfather must undergo general anesthesia, you can probably leave him in the hands of the staff once he's sedated. Before you leave, however, make a point of leaving a songbook on your grandfather's gurney and announcing clearly, "If granddaddy gets agitated, I suggest you start singing 'Home on the Range' or 'You Are My Sunshine.' Those are his favorites."

You're likely to get some startled looks from the staff, but keep a straight face. Get their attention and remind them that he has dementia, and that would be well-advised to fetch you as soon as he starts coming out of the anesthesia. It works every time!

(*See also:* Attitude; Baby Talk; Communication; Comprehension; Conversations; Empathy; Health; Humor; Laughter; Music; Singing)

■ ■ ■ ■ ■ ■ ■

Humor

Humor can help both of you over many of the bumps you experience in your daily lives. For example, your friend Fran has always had a good sense of humor, although now she has some difficulties with the language. Her jokes and funny sayings are sometimes a bit hard to understand, but you make a point of reacting to her little asides as you would expect her to react to yours. Occasionally, she misses the subtlety of some jokes, so try to be more obvious and basic with your amusing remarks. When you share a good laugh it can bring you closer together and give you some relief in situations that would otherwise be trying for both of you. Remember, you want to maintain her dignity at all times by making sure that you laugh with her, not at her.

You can use gross exaggerations, silly remarks, self-deprecation, or tell her stories about a faux pas of your own, real or fabricated. It will help her to hear that you make silly mistakes, too. You can always get a quick laugh by giving ridiculous choices (with a straight face, of course). For example, you can offer goofy choices at the ice cream parlor, "Which flavor would you like? Chocolate or salami?"

You can offer her silly choices when planning the day. For instance, you could say something like this: "Okay, we have two choices. You tell me what you want to do. We can spend the rest of the day at home sitting in our chairs staring into space and twiddling our thumbs, *or* we can go on an amazingly wonderful excursion to that new bookstore downtown followed by a cup of cappuccino at the coffee bar. I know this is a tough decision. Do you need some more time to think about it?"

Duh!

"Let's hit the road . . . but the road hasn't done anything, and besides, it would hurt us more than it would hurt the road. So maybe we should just drive on it instead."

"You look as happy as a clam! . . . By the way, how can you tell when a clam's happy?"

"I'm thinking, I'm thinking. Can't you hear the wheels turning? Hear that noise! Oh no, I guess that noise is a lawn mower. Oops!"

"Here we are, all belted into the car, ready to go; now if I can only find the keys. Have you noticed it helps to use keys when you drive a car?"

Offer Fran a piece of chocolate and very seriously explain to her how chocolate can improve her health, "Here's a piece of chocolate for you. Did I tell you that chocolate raises the endorphin level in our bodies? Endorphins are important for our immune systems and help keep us healthy. Now, you must think of this chocolate as medicine. You're not supposed to enjoy medicine, you know. You're not enjoying it, are you?"

(*See also*: Affection; Attitude; Empathy; Laughter)

H

I

■ ■ ■ ■ ■ ■ ■ ■

Identification

It's a good idea to get an identification bracelet for your wife that states her Alzheimer's condition, as well as any allergies she might have. Have it inscribed with her name, your address, and your phone number. It will help if strangers encounter her wandering about, or if they try to intervene and you need to quickly explain her situation to them.

Medical identifications are available as both bracelets and necklaces. Because a necklace might catch on something, a bracelet is the safer choice for ID for a confused person.

Ask about a medical alert bracelet at your local pharmacy, where you can find order forms, or check out the Resources section at the back of this book. The Alzheimer's Association has an excellent program named Safe Return, which combines ID bracelets with a hotline to facilitate uniting you with your Alzheimer's person when he or she has wandered off.

(*See also:* Aggression; Conversations; Safe Return)

■ ■ ■ ■ ■ ■ ■ ■

Incontinence

Since we were first potty trained, we've been conditioned to view urination and defecation as embarrassing or disgusting, even though they are functions as natural to the body as breathing. We've spent our lives being careful not to soil ourselves. From early infancy it's been drummed into our heads that we must use the toilet and wipe ourselves well. Your mother still has the same need to be clean, but sometimes doesn't remember until it's too late. It's important for her to continue using the toilet by herself as much as she can, even though she may become upset when she has an accident. Her short-term memory loss may actually be the cause, because she can no longer remember when she last used the bathroom. She doesn't think of it until her body has the urge, and by then it may be too late.

Your mother may understand and accept that she needs a panty shield, but she may still get upset and ashamed if she's had an accident. If you decide it's necessary to use incontinence aids, please call them "pads" or "briefs," never "diapers," a word that is demeaning to an adult. Also, although it may be inconvenient at times, you need to change her pad as soon as it is soiled.

You can establish a routine of taking her to the toilet frequently and at specific times: after meals, before leaving the house, before a nap or bedtime, and right after she gets up. You may need to accompany her to the toilet and coach her through the motions to make sure she actually relieves herself. It is also beneficial to learn her body language so that you can recognize the signs that she needs to use the toilet. She might suddenly seem distracted or perhaps she might start to twist in her seat.

When you are going to be away from home, it's a good idea to place a panty shield or pad in the crotch of her panties. If your mother's accidents become frequent, you may want to look into the variety of protective products available on the market. A heavy-duty panty shield or "half brief" may be all she needs. Keep in mind that most "full briefs" are taped in place at the waist and are almost impossible for an Alzheimer's person to remove by herself.

ACCIDENTS   Suppose your mother has just had an "accident" and she's distraught. You took her to the restroom after lunch, but now when you're coming out of the movies, you see that her pants have a wet spot. She's very agitated, complaining loudly that someone dressed her in the wrong pants, and she's rubbing at the spot frantically. In this situation, the best thing to do would be to calmly lead her to the restroom (which you notice always seems to be at the opposite end of the building).

Say to her, "Mom, I need to go to the bathroom so why don't you come with me. We brought along another pair of underwear so you can change into them and that'll make you feel so much better. This spot will dry really fast, and as soon as we get home, I'll help you change into another pair of pants."

While you take your time chatting with your mother along the way, you'll notice that as long as you stay calm, others will pay very little attention to the two of you. You're also letting your mom know by your tone and attitude that you care more about her than about any of the strangers around you. Don't rush her. When you get her to the toilet, you should remain cheerfully composed while you clean her up and help her change into clean underwear.

It may be an awkward maneuver for you with strangers all around, but maintain your nonchalant attitude while you change her half brief. It's easier to accomplish this while she's still sitting on the toilet. With the tiny stalls typical of public restrooms, you'll probably have to keep the door open to accommodate the two of you. Hopefully a handicap stall will be available, which will give you more privacy. Talk her through the motions in a normal tone of voice. This may be hard the first time, but remember that this is something that can happen to anybody and your only concern is for your mother's well-being. Other people in the restroom may surprise you with comments like, "I hope someone will be there for me like that when I need it!"

BEDTIME   Although your father uses the toilet by himself during the day, you still have to remind him to go. Even before it becomes a necessity, cover your dad's mattress with a full plastic sheet. Later, when it does become essential, place an underpad on top of the sheet. If possible, use a comforter in a cover instead of blankets and loose sheets. Blankets and sheets can become a tangled net for a confused person in a rush to reach the bathroom.

Most importantly, don't give your father anything to drink for the last two hours before his bedtime. Have him wear a half brief that can handle small accidents. Use them in place of his shorts because they pull on and off easily. When he's ready for bed, you'll probably still have to remind him to use the toilet sometime during the course of the night. If you're too late and he has an accident, reassure him in a kindly way. Say something like, "Oh well, anyone can have an accident, Dad." Talk cheerfully about something else while you change the sheets and his pajamas. Try to stay positive, even if it's three o'clock in the morning.

Your father may eventually need to advance to full briefs. (*Brief* is the accepted term for adult diaper.) There are a few brands featuring an elastic waistband, which can be pulled up or down like undershorts. The most widely sold full briefs are taped closed, which makes them just about impossible for your father to pull down or up by himself. If he wears them at night, he'll need your help to remove them in the morning.

PRODUCTS There's a bewildering variety of incontinence products on the market, from menstrual pads to full briefs. They basically fall into the following categories:

I

> Minimum protection: panty liners, panty shields

> Medium protection: half briefs, with elastic fasteners or elastic waistbands

> Maximum protection: full briefs, taped or with an elasticized waist for a more secure fit and ease of use for the Alzheimer's person

> Underpads: protection for beds, chairs, or car seats

These products are readily available at your local supermarket, drugstore, or membership store. Local home health stores and some mail-order houses sell more specialized versions.

(*See also:* Attitude; Bathroom; Communication; Dignity; Humor)

■ ■ ■ ■ ■ ■ ■ ■

Independence

Most of us would have a hard time giving up our independence. We equate our independence with self-respect and dignity. This is true of a person with dementia as well.

Suppose your uncle had been living in his own house before he came to live with you, when it became clear that he could no longer manage on his own. He's not happy with the arrangement. All his adult life he was self-employed and very much in control of every aspect of his own life, but now he's living in your house, by your rules and routines, so it's a very hard transition for him.

Because you've been conscious of this, you make sure that he has as much independence as possible. You continually give him choices and routinely ask for his opinions. You're trying to make him feel as if he has a part in making the day-to-day decisions. You can give him jurisdiction over his living area even if it's only his bedroom. Let him decide where and how things are arranged. When you have to clean it, try to do so either when he's not there, or ask him to help you, or offer to give him a hand. Say, "Hey Uncle Will, you said you'd like me to help clean your room. I can help you this afternoon; I hope that's all right with you."

If he's agreeable, you can act as his assistant. You can say something like, "I brought the vacuum cleaner. Would you like me to run it, or do you want to do it yourself?"

(*See also:* Dignity; Empathy; Personal Space; Privacy; Validation)

J

■ ■ ■ ■ ■ ■ ■ ■
Journals

You may want to keep a diary of your daily activities, even if it's only a line or two in a daybook. This will help you to keep track of your father's favorite meals and places to go, fun games, and entertaining stories. This is also a good way to record your dad's physical and mental conditions. Some medications have potentially serious side effects and the more information about his reactions that you can bring to his doctors, the better they'll be able to adjust the dose or find safer alternatives, if necessary.

If you enjoy writing, you can keep a journal of your father's stories or of amusing experiences you've shared. This will give you a priceless record of the time you spend together. When your father has moments of clarity, take advantage of them and encourage him to talk about his memories. You can encourage him to write an "autobiography" with your assistance. Augment it with your own notes. You may have heard his stories many times before, but they take on a special meaning when you write them down and they become part of your family chronicles.

(*See also:* Medication; Recording Memories)

K

■ ■ ■ ■ ■ ■ ■ ■

Kitchen

In most homes, the kitchen is the central meeting place and you probably spend a lot of time there. You'll want to find ways to safely include your Alzheimer's person in your daily activities there so that you won't have to leave him alone elsewhere in the house.

Your father never came near the kitchen during your growing-up years. As a matter of fact, he barely knew where it was, so when you suggest that he help you with the cooking, he may become incredulous. But since he's having trouble eating lately, you figure that this may be one way to get him interested in food again. Start by having him sit on a stool in the kitchen to watch you as you cook. Engage in a running commentary of the cooking process. Get him involved, one small step at a time. For example, you could say to him, "Dad, would you mind cutting up this banana for me? Small slices will be just fine, about a quarter of an inch."

Play it by ear and be sure he's using tools that are safe for him. Let him set his own pace as much as possible and allow his involvement to develop slowly. It's important that he enjoy himself, and who knows, his eating habits might even improve.

Your mother was known as quite a gourmet cook in her former social circle. But you were so intimidated by her skills that you stayed as far away from the kitchen as possible and missed out on learning some of her finest culinary tricks. Still, you've managed to become a fairly decent cook, even a subscriber to *Gourmet* magazine.

Your mother had several near disasters with fire and knives in her own kitchen while she was still living by herself, which is one of the reasons she's now living with you. Of course, it's been frustrating for her, because she has no memory of her accidents, so she thinks that you're just being mean or jealous by keeping her out of the kitchen.

Suppose your mom has been sitting with you in the kitchen while you cook, but she is driving you crazy with her constant comments. Nothing you do is done "her way," which, of course, in her mind, is the only right way. Before you explode in exasperation, consider getting her safely involved in the cooking process. Start by putting her in charge of the salads, cutting up soft fruits and vegetables, or mixing batters. Most importantly, ask her for her opinions and advice and listen patiently to her explanation, however jumbled and nonsensical it might be. In the end you'll do it your own way, but it will make her feel good to think you've followed her directions.

For instance, when you open a can of mushroom soup, you can say, "Mom, you used to make an incredible sauce for the roast chicken. I'd like to make it tonight. Let me see . . . I start by heating up the stock. Does this look right?"

K

She might respond with something like this: "They should be the right way. One, two, three, four. People think they can have two. That's right."

You will have no idea what she's talking about, but continue as if she is making perfect sense while you pretend to sprinkle seasonings into the pot: "and then I add these fresh herbs. Let me see . . . we have thyme and rosemary and your secret ingredient . . . What was it again?"

"Eight, nine, ten, eleven, twelve . . ."

"I think it's a dash of nutmeg, right? Twelve? I don't know. That sounds like too much. What do you think? Maybe it is two dashes. One, two. Oh yes, now that smells just like your famous sauce. You were always a marvelous cook, and I have so much to learn from you. Thank you so much for helping me out, Mom."

Since your mother likes to count these days, you can get her attention by counting with her, and you will make her feel good by paying her a compliment.

If your mom likes to fiddle around in the kitchen, you can set aside a drawer for her tools and the other kitchen utensils that she likes to work with. For cabinets that hold unsafe tools, use childproof safety locks.

Kitchen

You can also support her interest in cooking by helping her create her own recipe collection. Even if she's no longer able to cook on her own, she'll probably enjoy looking through your cooking magazines. You can encourage her to cut out recipes and paste them into a scrapbook. This can provide her with a diversion when you need it.

(*See also:* Fixations; Home Safety; Honesty; Loving Lies; Obsessive Behavior; Projects; Validation; Word Substitutions)

K

L

■ ■ ■ ■ ■ ■ ■

Laughter

Your cousin Emily will probably provide you with lots of hearty chuckles, but you don't want to make her self-conscious. Be sure to laugh with her, never at her, and try to find something in yourself that you can both laugh at, as well. Laughter will help ease your own stress and it also can help Emily to realize that you don't take her awkward mistakes seriously, so why should she?

Chocolate, exercise, hugs, and laughter raise the levels of endorphins in our bodies and boost our immune systems, so they're very powerful healing tools for both of you. Now that her thoughts are becoming more and more confusing, Emily will have a much easier time if you can help her approach daily life with a light heart and a sense of humor.

Since Emily's forgetting so much these days, she may enjoy the irony of you forgetting something too. When an occasion to laugh at yourself arises, say to Emily something like this: "You're not going to believe this, Emily. This morning, I couldn't remember where I had put my glasses. I looked all over the house for them. I even looked under my bed. Do you know where I found them? Right on top of my head! They were there all along, but I didn't realize it until I passed the mirror and saw my reflection out of the corner of my eye. Boy, did I laugh at myself!"

The best laughs come from your own experiences. Look back at your own life for funny stories. You can keep a log of the stories that really amuse Emily and bring her the most joy and then repeat them often, "Did I ever tell you about the . . ."

You can also start a collection of humorous books and videos, although that is probably easier said than done. Unfortunately, much contemporary adult humor tends to be mean-spirited. You might find some humorous books at the library, especially in the children's department. Also, look for classic movies and comedy videos.

(*See also:* Attitude; Empathy; Exercise; Games; Humor; Word Games)

■ ■ ■ ■ ■ ■ ■ ■

Listening

Your grandmother is delighted when you really "listen" to her. Her words don't make much sense to you, but by watching her body language and listening for verbal clues, you can get a sense of her intent. For example, if she says something like, "It is so grompsy, when they tool it," you can respond with something like, "It sounds as if you've given this matter a lot of thought."

She might glow with pleasure as she says, "That shilley is loyal, many now."

What's she talking about? You have no idea, but you can give her a neutral response like, "That's very interesting," to keep the conversational ball rolling. Then you might recall a TV program that she was watching with particular interest the night before. It's certainly worth a try, so you might say, "I think I heard them talking about that on TV last night." And who knows? She might happily agree with you.

By making these kinds of comments, you can find yourself engaged in a lengthy "discussion" with a totally delighted grandmother. Furthermore, giving her neutral responses might help you to eventually figure out what she's talking about.

Your friend Gertrude's still able to express herself in a somewhat linear fashion, but she's lost a lot of vocabulary so she uses replacement words. If you have some idea of what she means, you can use "active listening" to help her without sounding as if you're correcting her. For example, if she says, "The sessie's so much pretty. There was a well one," you might respond with, "Yes, I agree with you, Trudi. That was one of the nicest department stores we've been to in a long time. There was so much to look at. It sounds as if you particularly liked that beige sweater. Do you think we should go back and buy it?"

And if she becomes frustrated and dangles half-finished sentences, you can gently help her finish them as though finishing someone's sentences is a perfectly normal thing to do. For instance, if she says, "I want to go in . . . with the wheels." You might say with a smile, "The car? Funny you should say that, because I was just about to ask you if you wanted to go for a ride in the car later this afternoon. Great minds think alike, eh?"

(*See also:* Communication; Comprehension; Discussions; Normal; Validation; Word Substitutions)

■ ■ ■ ■ ■ ■ ■
Love

> *See:* Acceptance; Affection; Death and Dying; Loving Lies; Sexuality; Validation

L

■ ■ ■ ■ ■ ■ ■
Loving Lies

Alzheimer's disease starts by affecting the section of the brain that holds our short-term memory. As the disease progresses, more and more of stored memory is lost. It seems to be erased or fractured almost in a reverse mode, so that at one point, the only memories left somewhat intact are those from the earliest stages of life.

You may realize that your mother has slipped into an altered reality and at this moment she's thinking of herself as a little kid with her mother waiting at home. If you try to convince her that she's hallucinating, she might become unnecessarily upset. Instead you decide to "go into her reality." You use a loving lie.

Your mom was always a stickler for the truth, so you may have some qualms about lying to her. However, it might help you to remember that your lie is, in fact, her truth, because it is based on her reality at the moment. Called *therapeutic lies* by the geriatric community, this method is strongly advocated as an effective tool when working with Alzheimer's people, because it validates their realities. When you use a loving lie, you want to sound believable and sincere, and it's important to follow up a loving lie with some sort of diversion.

For example, suppose your mom's busy packing her all of her underwear into a shoebox. When you ask her what she's doing, she says, "Mother's waiting for me. I must go!" A useful response might be to say to her, "Oh, I'm sorry. I forgot to tell you. Your mother called and said she has a meeting at the church tonight and she wants you to stay here and eat dinner with me." And then, you could follow that up with a statement like this one, "You said earlier you wanted to help me fix dinner. If the offer still stands, I think now is a perfect time. Come, let's go to the kitchen."

Or imagine another time when your mother is very agitated and keeps repeating, "Someone stole my favorite beige coat! You just can't trust anybody these days!"

That beige coat had succumbed to the moths by the time you were fourteen, but you could calmly respond with, "We took it to the cleaners this morning. They said we can pick it up tomorrow. How about wearing your blue jacket today. You look so pretty in that color." Then divert her attention by saying, "I wonder if the new gardening magazine arrived yet. If you have time right now, would you mind checking the mail on the table?"

The loving lie should always sound authentic and in character. For example, your grandfather's friend obsesses about his wife's whereabouts, although she died eight years ago. Suppose someone tells him, "Oh, she went out shopping this afternoon." Rather than being reassured as expected, he may react with increased agitation. As it turns out, his wife had been a workaholic who had so little free time that shopping had become a special event reserved just for the two of them to spend some time together. When he's told that his wife has gone shopping without him, of course he becomes upset. That's why a loving lie must accurately reflect the circumstances of the people involved.

Loving Lies

Aunt Ellen was a long-standing member of a prominent civic organization. In spite of her shyness, she often made public appearances on its behalf. These events happened so long ago that you have no idea of what she's talking about when she asks you, "Where are my notes? What did I do with them? Have you seen them?"

You search her room and find a sheet of paper on her nightstand. But when you present it to her, this only seems to aggravate her further. You continue to search her room while you're searching your brain for a clue as to what she's talking about, when she says, "I can't go before them without my notes."

Ah! Your memory kicks in and you think, "A speech! She must be talking about a speech she gave." Remembering her occasional experiences as a public speaker, you sit down with her and seriously explain, "We got a telephone call while you were taking your nap. They called and said the event has been postponed until next week. The other two speakers have come down with that flu that's going around. So now you have a whole extra week to worry about it (ha, ha). If you want to rehearse, I'd be glad to be your guinea pig audience."

This is a perfect opportunity to encourage her to talk about her past experiences with civic affairs. Turn on your tape recorder, sit back, and listen. You might learn something new about Ellen at the same time that you're calming her down.

(*See also*: Communication; Diversions; Empathy; Normal; Reality; Validation)

L

Loving Lies

M

■ ■ ■ ■ ■ ■ ■
Massage

Your touch can be soothing to Dad when he's agitated. Simply resting your hand on his arm or back often can calm him. You share several hugs with him throughout the day and give him a casual back scratch now and then. You keep a bottle of lotion handy to massage his hands and, occasionally, his feet. Not only does this help to relieve the dryness in his skin, it is also the easiest way to soothe him and enhance his sense of connection to you.

A more elaborate massage can do wonders to make your father feel good, both physically and mentally. If he's shy because he's never had a massage before, use a gradual approach to help him feel more comfortable. Start by massaging his arms and legs until he becomes relaxed. After a while, ask him something like this, "It feels so good, doesn't it? Would you like to try a back massage?"

If he agrees, ask him to sit on a straight-back chair, facing backward, with his legs straddling the seat and his arms resting on the back of the chair. He can keep his shirt on for the first few times. As you stroke his back, describe what you are doing step-by-step.

Tell him, "I'm going to give you a good back massage, Dad. Can you feel how I'm rubbing your back? It's good for your muscles and your circulation. You'll feel so good after this. I guarantee it."

When you sense that he's feeling at ease, you can help him to remove his shirt as you explain what you are going to do. Reiterate how good it will feel. If he's shy, you can emphasize the "medical" necessity and physical benefits while you give him a back massage.

When both of you are ready, apply massage oil and lightly stroke his back in large circular moves. Do this very carefully, because elderly bones are fragile and elderly skin bruises easily. A deeper massage for your father would be best left to a professional. If he is feeling muscle pain or joint aches, it might be time to take him to a massage therapist with a specialty in geriatrics. Discuss this with his doctor before making a decision.

(*See also:* Affection; Empathy; Humor; Pain)

■ ■ ■ ■ ■ ■ ■ ■
Medication

Suppose your mother's doctor has suggested medications to improve her quality of life. Before you commit her to any of these medications, however, you'll want to investigate them thoroughly. Some of them may have very serious, possibly irreversible, side effects. You also may want to look into natural herbal remedies.

When you decide a medication is acceptable, keep a journal of your mom's mental and physical condition while she's on it. If you notice she is having a negative reaction, you may decide that you would be better off handling her conditions without using drugs, following instead the methods outlined in this book.

But suppose your mother has to be on "life-sustaining" medication. You want her to have the best results with the mildest side effects. So it would be an excellent idea to establish a rapport with your pharmacist and request circulars so you can discuss all of your mother's prescriptions and the possible alternatives.

There's an average of ten thousand prescription drugs on the market at any one time and each comes with a circular that describes the medication, benefits, side effects, test results, and so on, all, however, in the tiniest print. These circulars will be easier for you to read if you make copies of them enlarged at 200 percent.

There are also several excellent publications, written for the public, that review the most popularly prescribed medications. Check your local bookstore or library for these.

> **Tip!** Keep all medications and chemical substances (including cleaning liquids) securely locked up. Don't keep anything in the bathroom medicine cabinet or under the sink that your mother might mistakenly ingest (sweet-smelling liquid soaps, for example).

(*See also:* Alternative Remedies; Alzheimer's Medications; Dementia; Pain; Pills)

■ ■ ■ ■ ■ ■ ■
Memories

As the disease progresses, your grandmother will lose many of her recent memories or they will become so fractured that they won't make any sense to her. On the other hand, her childhood and early adulthood memories may still be pretty much intact. It's as though her life is a videotape that's being erased backward as the disease progresses. Your grandma may reach the point where she has no recollection of ever having been married or of having had any children. As she reaches back into the part of her memory that still makes sense to her, she's likely to confuse current family members with her siblings and her own parents.

For example, her grandson may look remarkably like her brother did at the same age, so when her grandson visits, she will greet him with a big smile and call him by her brother's name. Her grandson may look baffled and be at a loss for words because of the mix-up, but your grandmother's actions make perfect sense when you take into consideration how Alzheimer's is affecting her short-term memory.

COACHING   Coaching often helps an Alzheimer's person to remember stories and details that he or she might otherwise forget. For example, after a visit to another family member, you might say something like this to your father: "Dad, when we visited your sister yesterday, the two of you talked a lot about growing up together. You had such a good time talking to each other and remembering all the old stories." Then reiterate as much of their conversation as you can in order to encourage his participation. This might lead him to join in with you because he won't feel pressure to remember anything specific, so his memory might flow more easily.

At this point, and with great enthusiasm, he will once again regale you with the same old favorite story. Telling this anecdote brings him such joy, but you fear that you may not be able suppress a howl of "God spare us! Not again." Instead of feigning interest yet one more time, wait for a lull in his story and then try to redirect him by asking a question that might stimulate a new aspect of the same old saga. For example, say, "I really enjoy hearing about your experiences with your sister. I was wondering if the two of you played the same games that I played when I was a kid. Did you play hide and seek? . . . or how about (name a game that he saw you play when you were a child)?"

This could trigger additional stories, although his oft-repeated tale may be the only one about his sister that's still in his memory bank. If that's the case, you might instead ask a question so general that he won't feel put on the spot. For instance, you could ask, "Did you have to walk a long way to school when you were a kid, Dad?" This is a pretty safe question, because practically everyone of his generation walked to school.

Or you might initiate a conversation about a memory from your shared past. "Do you know what I really miss? Listening to the radio with you and Mom when I was little. There was one particular show we all loved to listen to. What was the name of it? Darn it, I don't remember, do you?"

It can be reassuring for your father to hear that you occasionally have problems remembering things too. No matter what he recalls, just go along with him, although there's a good chance he'll remember the name of a radio show more easily than his mother's birthplace. You may have been thinking of *The Shadow*, but if he says *The Jack Benny Show*, it doesn't really matter. The important thing is that the two of you can reminisce about good times you've shared.

PITFALLS   You want to stay away from challenging your father's memory with questions that require specific recollection. That means it's probably best to avoid questions like these: "How many children do you have?" "Where did you live?" and "How old were you?"

You may find it disturbing that your father can't even remember his own children but you'll find that if you force the issue, you'll only make him depressed and unhappy.

"Don't you remember . . . ?" and "Do you remember . . . ?" are questions that may trigger a panic in him when he realizes that he can't remember and he thinks he ought to. In other words, these kinds of questions emphasize his dementia to him.

Instead, you can start his reminiscing by recounting an event or person. Go into details until you sense recognition on his part. "It was some time ago, so you may not remember." Or you could say, "You met this person months ago and there were a lot of other people around at the time, so I'd be surprised if you'd remember." In that way, you give your father an opening and take some of the pressure off him.

EXCEPTIONS Questions like, "Did you have a favorite subject in school?" or "Did you enjoy Halloween?" or "Did you like Ford Model Ts?" are such broad subjects that he's apt to remember something, and if he doesn't offer a response, it doesn't matter because even he is aware that this is inconsequential chitchat.

(*See also:* Communication; Listening; Normal; Questions; Recording Memories; Validation)

M

■ ■ ■ ■ ■ ■ ■ ■

Money

Money was an important symbol of your friend Arthur's self-respect throughout his productive adult life. You've been handling his money for some time now, but you give him a few bills and some change to keep in his wallet so he can pay for small purchases now and then.

Suppose one day the two of you are standing at the checkout stand in a supermarket when he looks at the few bills in his wallet and becomes very agitated. He says, "Who took my money? Someone took my money! I had all my money in here. Now it's gone. Who took all my money?"

Take his arm gently and say, "May I see your wallet, Art? I see . . . looks like you have about fifteen dollars. I think that's all you decided to bring today. Yesterday you put the rest of your money in the bank for safekeeping."

"I don't remember doing that."

"Yesterday was such a busy day, I had also forgotten about the bank until you brought it up just now. I'll go ahead and pay our bill and you can pay me back later when we go back to the bank, okay?"

If Arthur keeps obsessing about his money, you can arrange to have him receive a "paycheck" in the mail every Friday. It will be a wonderful ego booster for him. You can then offer to "deposit" his "check" at the bank and later tear it up.

———————————

Your friend Patty loves carrying her purse. She often fills it with an odd assortment of things: a tube of toothpaste, some old greeting cards, and a solitary sock. Sometimes you slip a few bills into her wallet before taking her out.

Imagine you've just finished lunch at a local café. Patty insists on treating you, but you've forgotten to give her some money today. It might be tempting to remind her just how well you have been handling her bank account all these years, but you resist. Say, instead, "Oh, Patty, I couldn't let you do that. You treated the last time we went to lunch, so now it's my turn."

You can take advantage of the situation and give her a compliment that will help to divert her attention: "You're such a generous person. I'm so lucky to be your friend. You have taught me so much with your many examples of kindness."

(*See also:* Diversions; Independence; Loving Lies)

■ ■ ■ ■ ■ ■ ■ ■
Movies

There's something special about watching a film in a theater with a large screen and big sound. Your mother may not be able to follow the story line, but don't be surprised if she reacts to the overall "quality" of the picture. If the characters are well written and the actors convincing, she will likely enjoy the experience, even if she doesn't remember the plot. Most of us forget the plots of many of the movies we've enjoyed; your mother just forgets a lot sooner—like the moment she leaves the theater.

M

Going to the movies has always been a favorite pastime of yours and you've missed it since your mom's been living with you. Imagine that one afternoon you can't find someone to stay with your mother so you decide to take her to the movies with you, although you're worried that she won't be able to follow the story line and might not enjoy it. She's felt anxious in crowded places lately, so you feel concerned, even as you buy the matinee tickets.

Your mother, however, is quite excited as she walks into the theater lobby. After a trip to the restroom, you make your way to your seats in the nearly empty theater. The previews confuse her, so you may have to remind her that the movie hasn't started yet.

When the movie finally begins, you discreetly observe her while she watches it and you are pleasantly surprised at her attention. She's enjoying this! Afterward, when you try to talk about the plot, she has no idea of what you're talking about, and yet, when you ask her if she liked going to the movie and would she like to come back, she responds in enthusiastic agreement.

Your mother may have a hard time following a movie on a small television screen with all the distractions that are present in a home setting, but a movie theater is an exciting and magical place that may command her full attention. Select movies that you yourself want to see. Your enjoyment will likely rub off on your mom.

(*See also:* Comprehension; Reality)

■ ■ ■ ■ ■ ■ ■ ■

Music

Music can bring joy, peace, and positive energy, or it can put you into a state of aggravation or nervousness. In the lives of human beings, music is so powerful that the sense of music is apparently the first sense we grasp, even while still in the womb, and it is the last of our senses to go. You want to keep that in mind when you come to the point of helping your husband through the last days of his life. Play his favorite music to help him feel at peace.

The use of music can be a great addition to your daily routines. There is a wide variety of music available that's designed to aid in mood relaxation and elevation. If your husband is agitated, try playing one of these tapes or CDs in the background while you try to figure out what's bothering him. You can use mellow music to help him relax before bedtime and you can use nostalgic big band music to elevate his mood when he's blue and feeling down.

———————————

Imagine you've invited a few friends to a small dinner party, the first sort of formal event you've hosted since your Aunt Lisa has been living with you. She's been doing her best to be of help in the kitchen all afternoon, but you're so used to cooking alone that you spend most of your time trying to find something for her to do. After a few hours of this, your dinner is running late, you're feeling testy, and Lisa is quite agitated. In your calmest voice you try to tell her that you have everything under control, but she reacts, feeling obviously rejected. She feels useless and is close to tears.

Having run out of projects in the kitchen, walk her into the dining room while you try to convince her that she's the only one who could possibly set the table to perfection. She grumbles, and mumbles in protest: "You just don't like my cooking, do you? I remember when you were a little kid, you'd spit out your food. I just can't do anything right, can I? I hate it here. I'm going back home tomorrow!"

You do your best to stay calm through this tirade. You must admit that it hurts. You know that arguing with her is hopeless, so instead you turn to the stereo, play one of the Chopin CDs you had chosen for the evening, and return to the kitchen, leaving Lisa to her angry protesting. After a few minutes you realize she's quiet, so you sneak a peek and see her sitting in the big easy chair in front of the stereo. Her eyes are closed and she has a faint smile on her face. She's positively beatific sitting there. As you silently thank Chopin and his colleagues and return to chopping the garlic, you make a mental note yourself that you just remembered how powerful music can be.

———————————

Suppose your father has been having bouts of depression and loneliness. At times he hallucinates that your mother is waiting for him, and when you tell him she's been dead for fifteen years, he either gets angry or he withdraws and won't eat. You've discovered that the "cure" to this miserable state is to play his collection of

M

oldies like Glenn Miller and Duke Ellington as background music while you sit with him for a few minutes and listen to him talk about the early days with your mother. Then follow up the sound of the big bands with the gentle sounds of Brahms, so by the time bedtime comes around, you will both be feeling mellow and ready for a restful and contented sleep.

(*See also*: Death and Dying; Exercise; Hospital; Singing)

M

N

■ ■ ■ ■ ■ ■ ■ ■
Neighborhood Flyer

Wandering is a common phenomenon in Alzheimer's people. It can rightfully cause a lot of anxiety in caregivers. If this is one of your problems, there are some precautions you can take.

For example, suppose your mother has started to wander. The other day the two of you were separated at the mall. You were beside yourself with worry until a security guard located her. Since that occurrence, you have posted signs on your exits: "Do Not Go Out This Door" and you've ordered an identification bracelet for her. Even with these precautions, there's still a possibility that she'll wander off. Your mother looks perfectly normal, so it's not obvious to strangers that she may need help.

If you live on a typical street or in an apartment building, you may be acquainted with your immediate neighbors, but probably few people beyond those. Still, the neighborhood has often come together to help look for a lost dog or cat. It may be worth distributing a flyer to alert the neighborhood of her condition. You can make up your own or use our example on the following page.

(*See also:* Identification; Safe Return; Wandering)

Mom's Picture

Mom's name and description

Dear Neighbor,

My mother and I live in your neighborhood. Mother has Alzheimer's disease and is often very confused. If you see her alone on the street, please help us in one of the following ways:

Mom wears a medical alert bracelet with our phone number.

If we don't answer the phone, we're out looking for her. Please leave your phone number and address on our voice mail and we will be right over to get her.

If you're not comfortable with any of the above, please call the police right away with the location where you last saw her and the direction in which she was headed.

We realize this may be an imposition and we appreciate in advance any assistance you give us.

Thank you,

Your name

P.S. Mom likes strawberry jam, tea with a half teaspoon of sugar, ice cream, and potato chips. She loves children and cats.

Neighborhood Flyer

■ ■ ■ ■ ■ ■ ■

Normal

Your sister's behavior may seem odd to you at times, but keep in mind that she still thinks of herself as normal. From her point of view, it's the circumstances that are strange and she's merely reacting to them. You can help her maintain her self-confidence by addressing her with a normal attitude and tone of voice.

This feeling of "normal" is at the core of our self-awareness. We are all different, of course, and can only view the world from our individual perspectives, which are shaped by genetics, environment, and culture. If you were to ask your sister, she might acknowledge a bit of a memory problem, but other than that she considers herself perfectly normal.

"But she seems so normal." You've gotten used to hearing this when people learn that your sister's been diagnosed with Alzheimer's disease. Wouldn't you still consider yourself normal if you had a broken arm, missing teeth, arthritis, or diabetes? Now, how about baldness, hearing impairment, or sight impairment? So why should you feel any different about Alzheimer's? We all think of ourselves as normal, including the memory-impaired. Your sister has Alzheimer's disease, but she's not "sick" as such. Rather, she's in an altered state of mind and is not cognizant of the dramatic changes in her personality. However, the world does feel more and more confusing to her.

Suppose one day your sister gets lost going to the bathroom after having had no problems for months. She has suddenly lapsed into a different reality and she's back in her childhood home where the bathroom was at the opposite end of the house. In her mind she's normal, but the bathroom location has changed. You can help her by relating to the "normal" in her and by acknowledging her reality. Let her know that forgetting can happen to anybody.

She might say, "Where is it? I can't find it, they moved it. Where's the bathroom?"

And you can respond by saying, "Come with me, I'll be glad to show you. I think I know how you feel. Sometimes I wake up in the morning and everything looks weird to me because I was dreaming about my old house right before I woke up. It's such a strange feeling, isn't it? But rest assured, the bathroom is right down this hallway."

N

You can reassure her by asking for her suggestions on things that don't tax her memory. You can make up a "problem" and ask her advice on gardening, cooking, or relationships. She might just surprise you. She may have lost a lot of her memory, but her core personality hasn't changed, and to some degree her common sense is still there. It's important to her self-confidence that you value her opinion, whether or not you choose to follow her advice.

(*See also:* Empathy; Loving Lies; Questions; Transitions; Validation)

N

Normal

O

■ ■ ■ ■ ■ ■ ■ ■

Obsessive Behavior

Some Alzheimer's people develop obsessions. One possible explanation for this may be that they're trying to bring order into the confusion of their world. Sometimes the obsessions will start up suddenly when there's a major change in their lives. The cause could also be physical discomfort, such as an ingrown toenail or an illness, as well as a change in the person's environment or a new person in the household.

Your aunt Frieda has developed an obsession with counting. You've taken her to the doctor for her health checkups and everything seems to be in order. There is nothing wrong with her counting, and in fact, it seems to bring her some kind of peace. She will count the steps when you walk with her and she'll count when you help her to get dressed. She starts counting whenever she's not engaged in conversation or an activity. Rather than allowing yourself to become exasperated by this repetitive numbers game, try to join in cheerfully: "Do you think we'll reach a hundred before we get to the door? I bet we will. You're already at eighty-four, aren't you? Eighty-five, eighty-six, . . . Boy, you're way ahead of me. But I trust your judgment. I remember when I was a kid, you'd help me with my math. I wonder if I would have learned any of it if it hadn't been for you."

(*See also:* Diversions; Fixations; Kitchen; Signs; Word Substitutions)

■ ■ ■ ■ ■ ■ ■ ■

Outings

It does your husband a lot of good to get out. He may not remember exactly where you went, but he seems rejuvenated and more relaxed when you get home. Later at dinner you can tell him the "story" of your day. He may remember some of it and chime in. If he doesn't, he's simply hearing what a wonderful time you both had.

The last time you really explored your community was during the elementary school field trips you took when you were nine or ten years old. Lately, the two of you have been visiting museums, galleries, libraries, and parks. You aim for one outing a week, often going back to favorite haunts.

DRIVES   Imagine that you had planned to take your wife to the library today, but now you realize that there just isn't enough time. She's getting restless, so you decide to take her for a short drive instead. Say something like this, "Sweetie, I'm getting cabin fever. I need to get out of here. How about you? Wanna go for a drive with me?"

Your trip doesn't have to be a long one to be enjoyable. You can take a leisurely drive around the neighborhood and talk about what you see along the way: grass that's too high and needs cutting, big blue flowers or small yellow ones, a cute little dog, or a garbage truck making its rounds. Cruise along with a relaxed and carefree attitude. Your wife may be happily chatting, and although she may not be making much sense, go along with her conversation enthusiastically. Once in a while let your wife decide where to go. As you get ready to pull out into the street, ask her to point in which direction you should drive. Say, "Okay Honey, which way do we go?"

When you approach the first major intersection ask her again, "Now, when we get to the light, do we go this way or that? Or straight ahead?"

You may end up driving in circles, but so what? At least it's not boring and your wife may feel empowered by making the decisions. Keep it up for as long as she enjoys it, although it's likely that she'll tire soon. When you get home and talk about your outing, you can honestly give her the credit for an enjoyable trip.

You can say to her, "Wow, what a trip! It was so much fun having you lead the way. I had a great time. I got to see streets I didn't even know existed. We saw all those beautiful flowers. They reminded me of our garden. Except I think your flowers are much prettier. You've always been such a great gardener."

Your wife may love to listen to you talk about your life together when you include stories about her. She may not be able to remember specific events, so avoid asking her directly: "Do you remember. . . ?" Instead, try a storytelling approach:

"Speaking of flowers, do you know what one of my earliest memories about the two of us is? It's the time when I decided to 'help' you with the tulips, and I did it all wrong. You were so sweet. You thanked me and you didn't even get mad. I mean, I had just ruined your finest flower bed! Every time I see a tulip, that memory comes back to me. You know how I'm always adopting half-wilted plants at the store to save them from certain death. Do you suspect that I'm trying to make up for what I did to your tulips?"

GALLERIES   Your friend Betty always loved art shows, so you explore local art museums and galleries on your outings with her. When you find a gallery that Betty's particularly fond of, talk to the staff about her dementia. The next time you visit, the staff's recognition of her can make her feel knowledgeable and important.

If you visit a gallery in the morning, you can usually have the place to yourselves, which will give the two of you plenty of time to talk about the art. Ask the gallery director for announcements or flyers of past shows that you can use later for collage projects, or perhaps Betty can glue them into one of her scrapbooks.

LIBRARIES   Your mother still thinks of herself as an avid reader, although she usually doesn't get past the first page, which she happily reads over and over again. A trip to the library can become a favorite outing and help to fill her day.

If she loves gardens, find her a beautiful picture book of flowers, but be sure to open it to a picture, or she might not get past the opening text. This also would be a good time to reminisce with her. She probably remembers working in her own garden. If she doesn't, you can still entertain yourselves by creating richly detailed stories about fantasy gardens.

While you are at the library, check out some music books for your sing-alongs, how-to books for crafts projects, and books of poetry and short stories to read aloud. In addition, many libraries have excellent video collections available for checkout, with selections from *National Geographic* and PBS: They stock many shows like *Masterpiece Theater* or documentaries about nature. Most libraries also carry books on tape, which your mother might enjoy if she can still follow a good story line.

MUSEUMS   You and your father have discovered a local museum that offers free admission to seniors one day a week. Fortunately, wheelchairs are available, so when your dad is tired, you can wheel him around. Say, "Aren't we lucky? Here's a wheelchair we can use. Oh, I know you don't really need it, but this is such a big place and there's so much to see. This way you don't have to waste your energy on walking around."

Wheel him to those exhibits you are sure will particularly interest him. You may end up looking at only one exhibit the entire afternoon. Often, we feel the pressure to look at every single thing in a museum, so at first you may become restless with such a limited approach. Remember, you're there for sheer pleasure, so do what feels right to your father.

PICNICS   You and your brother Ben often talk about the wonderful annual family picnics of your childhood. Of course, during the reminiscing only the pleasures are remembered, like Grandma's potato salad, Aunt Ella's peach pie, and the softball games. Miraculously forgotten are the ants, flies, and running for cover from cloudbursts. In Ben's mind a picnic s still the ultimate outing, so the two of you can have a lot of good times making picnic plans. On your drives you often look for perfect picnic locations.

One beautiful summer day, you fill your picnic basket with a checkered tablecloth and a couple of brightly colored plastic plates, but you pack only a bottle of juice and a few crackers, because you want to make the picnic short and sweet. Aside from the usual dis-comforts of bugs and wind, picnic benches are uncomfortable and often very hard on elderly bottoms.

All too often the idea of a picnic is far more fun than the real thing, but a short ten-minute picnic can provide you with hours of reminiscing later. When you drive past your picnic location on later drives, you can relive it by saying, "Look, Ben, there's our favorite picnic bench in the shade of that big tree. We had such a good time there, we should have another picnic soon, don't you think?"

The next picnic may not take place until next summer, but you can still talk about it and plan for it in the meantime. Use the idea of picnics in your fantasy games on cold winter days when you are housebound. Get as elaborate as you can in your descriptions as you "plan" and encourage Ben to come up with ideas. Often, these talks about favorite activities can lead to joyful reminiscing on his part, so have your tape recorder handy.

SHOPPING   Dad gets tired and overloaded easily, so you keep your shopping simple. By now, you've learned to adjust your pace to his. Nowadays, you find yourself actually enjoying taking life a little slower. Little did you know that you could take such pleasure in going to the hardware store, but your father takes you on a tour with detailed explanations of the numerous bins of bolts, nails, and tools. He may be confused at home, but here, in his element, he has his old confidence back. The hardware store is his old stomping ground and you can listen with delight to the man you used to know. There may be days when you are the last "customers" to leave.

It may take visits to three or four different hardware stores before you find one with a staff and an owner who will encourage you to browse without asking you to spend a dime. You might even get several members of the staff to take time to "talk shop" with Dad, and the owner might give him expired catalogs for his workshop at home.

O

Perhaps you and your friend Susie have been going to the mall together for years, usually spending the better part of the day window-shopping. Susie especially likes to browse at a few of her favorite shops and then stop for lunch in the food court. These outings have always been fun for you both and you've reorganized your life to accomplish shopping for most clothes and other nonfood items on these trips.

Susie takes special delight in helping you with your clothing selections, but occasionally she wants you to buy something that you definitely don't want. When you are at the register, you can replace it with your choice, but do it when she's not looking so her feelings won't be hurt. Allowing Susie help choose your clothes may make it more acceptable to her when you make choices about her outfits.

Your local supermarket may have wheelchairs with small shopping baskets. As long as you don't need to do major shopping, the basket has plenty of room. You and Susie can have a fulfilling adventure at the supermarket, even if it's only to buy one particular item, like a box of bath salts or a basket of strawberries. While at the supermarket, explore something that's new to you: Greek stuffed grape leaves if you're Norwegian; Swedish meatballs if you're Indonesian. Or you and Susie can count the number of different brands of canned peas. You'll find that it doesn't really matter what you're looking at as long as you are sharing the experience.

After you get home you can talk about your experiences and some of the things you saw. She may not remember much about your outing, but that really doesn't matter. What's important is that she hears that you enjoyed her company and that you're pleased with her purchase. And, on a positive note, the new bath salts may make bath time more enjoyable for her. Say to her, "We had a good time this morning when we went to the market. It'll be fun to try your new bath salts. I bet that apple scent is going to make a nice bath. I think we should try it out right now, don't you?"

(See also: Activities; Bath Time; Conversations; Crowds; Discussions; Identification; Personal Space; Projects; Restaurants; Safe Return; Walking; Wandering)

P

■ ■ ■ ■ ■ ■ ■ ■
Pacing

Pacing is a common behavior in Alzheimer's people. When it occurs late in the day, it's known as "sundowning." Your grandfather may have an uncontrollable physical need to move, so you can help him by making sure that he has a safe path on which to pace, as well as plenty of liquids to drink so he won't become dehydrated.

Imagine that your grandfather has started to pace. He makes the rounds of your house by cruising down the hallway, goes through the kitchen down to the living room, and then back to the hall to start the cycle all over again. It's distracting as well as distressing for you. Usually, you can guide him to his personal space and get him started on a project. He's very cooperative and stays for a few minutes, but then he resumes his rounds. If this is the case, weather permitting, you can take him for a walk around the block. This will likely help him to calm down, and the exercise will be good for both of you.

Of course, his pacing may be psychological in nature. For example, he may feel he's neglected to do something but he can't quite think of what it was, so he paces to try to remember. This can be especially hard on him if he used to be an active person. He might need some mental stimulation to help him focus. Consider setting up a work space for him that will relate to his former job or career.

If he is on medication and his pacing is a sudden development, talk to his doctor as soon as possible. Certain medications can cause physiological problems. His doctor can tell you about alternatives to the medication that might be causing him trouble.

(*See also:* Agitation; Diversions; Personal Space; Projects; Sundowning)

■ ■ ■ ■ ■ ■ ■

Pain

Because of her dementia, your cousin Rhoda sometimes forgets that she's got an injury or a sore until it hurts her again. It's your natural inclination to comfort her if she feels a twinge in her bruised back and reacts by whimpering like a baby. With great solicitude in your voice you might say to her, "Oh, Rhoda, your back's hurting you again, isn't it?"

Unfortunately, while showing her that you're concerned, you may have also unintentionally told her two things that she had completely forgotten because of her dementia: (1) that her back is hurt, and (2) by the tone of your voice, that her injury must be serious. You will help her more by maintaining a positive demeanor and not allowing any worry to show in your voice. Instead, while she is reacting to the twinge you might say, "Rhoda, let me help you sit up straight again so you can feel better."

Perhaps Rhoda has a nasty cut on the back of her hand and it's time to change the dressing and reapply ointment. When you remove the bandage, it might be painful to her, so soften the dressing by applying warm water with a cotton ball. Carefully explain to her in your "coaching" voice what you're going to do. Say, "Rhoda, we have to change your bandage. You cut yourself and I have to put more ointment and a new bandage on it so it can heal. Do you want to pull it off yourself? Or do you want me to do it?"

She may start to remove the bandage but she'll probably wind up letting you do it in the end. Say to her, "I'll pull it off as gently as I can. I hope it won't hurt too much." Your cousin will handle it best if you explain everything that you're doing and why. Note that she may need to hear you repeat that information many times.

Remember that because of her dementia, she has no recollection of her injury, so as soon as you make her more comfortable, she will forget about the pain.

(*See also:* Affection; Coaching; Diversions; Empathy; Health; Humor)

■ ■ ■ ■ ■ ■ ■ ■
Paperwork

The following personal papers should be with your mother at all times:

> Her social security number, Medicare, Medicaid, and other insurance information

> List of emergency contact numbers

> Copy of her durable power of attorney for financial matters

> Copy of your mother's health care power of attorney, which includes a living will

> Copy of your mother's DNR (do not resuscitate) order

The durable power of attorney for financial matters is a notarized document that gives you the legal right to make financial and property decisions on your mother's behalf.

The health care power of attorney (HCPOA) is a signed document stating your mother's choices of the person(s) who will make health-care choices for her if she's unable. This document usually includes provisions addressing the withdrawal of medical treatment if she has a terminal or incurable illness. (It is also known as a living will.)

A DNR (do not resuscitate) order is a signed document stating that your mother does not want to receive CPR (cardiopulmonary resuscitation) in the event her heart stops. Discuss this with her doctor and, if you decide to establish a DNR order for her, keep it with her at all times. CPR is rarely what we see on television or in the movies. In reality it's successful only some of the time. It can be extremely aggressive, often causing broken ribs and a crushed breastbone. Is this something you want to subject your mother to? Ask a local EMT (emergency medical technician), fire department, or hospital for a copy of their standard DNR order form. If you want your mother's wishes to be respected, it's crucial for this document to be instantly recognizable by any emergency personnel in your area.

P

Be sure to keep copies of your mother's HCPOA and DNR forms at all of her doctors' offices, at her adult day-care center, and with any family members or friends with whom she spends time.

If your mom has started wandering, create a personal information sheet, which should include highlights of her background to help her rescuers relate to her; add a recent 5 x 7 or 8 x 10 photograph (or a photocopy of one) of her, and take copies of both to your local police department. They should keep them on file in case they should find your mom wandering. She should wear her medical alert identification bracelet at all times.

(*See also:* Identification; Neighborhood Flyer; Safe Return; Wandering)

■ ■ ■ ■ ■ ■ ■ ■
Personal Space

When you set aside an area in your home specifically for your friend who has Alzheimer's, you're letting her know that her needs are as important as your own. Her own personal space will help to give her a sense of purpose. Fill it with objects relating to her favorite activities. Then when you need a diversion for her, you can steer her into her own space and help her get started on a project.

Your friend took great pride in her apartment and spent hours cleaning and arranging her things. It was very hard on her to give it up and have to share a house with you. Of course, you've been doing your best to help her feel at home, and her own room is filled with her things. But you don't want her to spend her days squirreled away in her bedroom all day, so you've hung some of her pictures on the living room walls and displayed a few of her knickknacks among yours.

Another possible solution to make her feel more at home is to give her a daytime space of her own. It could be an entire room or just a corner of your workroom or kitchen. The size of her personal space is less important than the feeling of having her own personal domain.

OFFICE   Your uncle Fred ran his own company and retired a long time ago, but he's been quite confused lately, thinking he's still a working man. You've tried to convince him that he's lucky to be a retired man of leisure, but he's often miserable. He feels useless and gets angry, and frequently insists that he must go to the office. When you try to tell him that he sold the business several years ago, that only makes him more agitated.

Suppose that one day you find some paperwork from his old company. It's a challenge for you to figure out which pieces of paper are "real" business documents to him, but you finally sort through them all. Make copies of the paperwork that will help you to launch his new "office" in the corner of the kitchen where he keeps all his files, invoices, and notebooks.

With his own office to go to, he'll spend hours, sorting out papers and making copious notes in his date book. At the end of his "workday," whether it lasts thirty minutes or three hours, try to make time for him and listen to his business plans and analyses. After telling you all about it, he can then get on with the day, feeling a sense of accomplishment.

At one time in her life your mother was a busy and successful buyer for a well-known women's clothing chain, so these days it's difficult for her to be idle. She often gets moody and restless in the late afternoon, which was the time when she used to close the books at the end of the business day.

She needs to get back to "work," so set up a desk for her in a corner of your home. Scout around the local office supply store for order forms, tally sheets, in and out baskets, a pencil caddy, paperclips, markers, highlighters, and so on. Buy subscriptions to a few fashion magazines, get on the mailing lists of fashion catalogs, and collect fabric swatches.

Once she starts "going to work" every afternoon with great determination, you are careful to respect her space. For instance, when you want her attention, say, "Excuse me, Mom, I'm sorry to interrupt. I'm making some coffee and I was wondering if you're ready for a break?" At dinner, the two of you can share the details of your day: Ask her, "How was your day? Did you get those orders done?"

Personal Space

You can browse boutiques together. It's likely you'll be impressed with her knowledge and clarity as you watch her scrutinizing styles, workmanship, and details. She may be very forgetful about other things, but she's quite lucid on these excursions. These times together are precious and it would be a good idea to keep a journal of your experiences.

STUDIO   Your grandmother fancied herself an artist when you were a child. She took classes in oil painting and watercolor techniques, and she had a small easel set up in the corner of her laundry room. Although nothing ever came of it, her artistic yearnings have never diminished.

Grandma's been living with you for some time now. You go to galleries together and have had a lot of fun with collages and other craft projects. However, her dementia is getting worse and she's often agitated and restless. It helps her to create something. Set up projects that she can handle on her own without requiring your participation, other than a word of encouragement now and then.

You can set up a "studio" space for her. Keep it small (a big studio can be too intimidating), with an easel, a canvas, and some basic supplies. Even if she's no longer able to create without your help, when she's surrounded by items that remind her of some of her happiest times, she might be happy arranging and rearranging her supplies. Also, ask your local art supply store for old cast-off stuff, such as dried-up paint tubes.

You can also expand on your grandmother's projects by helping her do research on different artists or maintain files of art catalogs or scrapbooks with announcements, if she enjoys that sort of activity. Whenever she gets restless and needs a diversion, you can direct her to the studio. Note that it's important for you to treat her endeavors seriously.

In her personal "studio," encourage your grandmother to talk about her work and listen with sincerity. No matter what she's created, you can support her by commenting on her choices of colors, shapes, or composition. Don't gush over anything she has created unless you mean it. She's likely to be aware if you're faking it. Instead ask her questions you know she can answer; for example, say something neutral like, "I notice that you're using a lot of blue in your paintings. That's your favorite color, isn't it?"

Most of all, don't presume that you know what it is she's painted. Don't say, "What's that supposed to be? A house?" unless you're absolutely sure that it really is a house. If your grandmother used to be a good artist but has now lost her painting skills, it might hurt her feelings to think that you can't recognize what she's painted.

WORKSHOP   When you were a kid, your father was always tinkering with one project or another in his beloved workshop. He had all kinds of tools then, although now you know he's not able to handle tools safely anymore.

Dad's been getting restless and has started pacing, so you set up a "shop" for him in the garage. Ask the local hardware store for some outdated catalogs and check out garage sales and flea markets for odds and ends in nuts, bolts, hooks, and other hardware items.

The next time your father starts pacing, you can redirect him to his personal space: Say, "Did you find that tool you were looking for? What was it? A router?"

He just might disappear into his "shop" and return a few minutes later with an armload of woodworking catalogs, and an answer to your query. "No, of course not, I already have a router. Now where's that catalog? Come here, I'll show you."

Sit down with him and look at the catalogs together as he describes one tool after another. You may find yourself caught up in his explanations and asking questions in earnest. When he's talking "shop," he's the father you remember, knowledgeable and wise, with very little of his dementia in evidence.

(*See also:* Activities; Diversions; Exercise; Gardening; Kitchen; Outings)

■ ■ ■ ■ ■ ■ ■

Pets

It has long been recognized that animals have a positive therapeutic effect for most people. Just stroking a dog or a cat can lower the stress level and blood pressure. More progressive nursing homes are even employing furry "pet therapists," because of their soothing effects on the residents. Cats, dogs, and rabbits are favorites.

Imagine that one day when you arrive early at the day care center to pick up your grandmother, you find her totally engrossed in a small dog that had been brought to visit by the local animal shelter volunteer. She's gently stroking the dog, a smile beaming on her face, making her look peaceful and happy. You'd once considered adopting a cat or a dog, but were concerned that it would be too much for her. Watching her enjoyment makes you reconsider the possibility.

You can contact your local shelter and ask them to keep an eye out for a sweet and gentle cat or dog for your grandmother to adopt. Puppies and kittens are adorable, but they are frisky and may be harder for her to handle, so it's probably a better idea to get an adult pet.

If your landlord does not permit pets, consider setting up a fish tank. Many people find it soothing and very calming just to watch the fish swim by. Some educational toy stores sell a fake aquarium that is so realistic that your grandmother may try to feed the fish.

(*See also:* Affection)

P ■ ■ ■ ■ ■ ■ ■ ■
Pills

Your mother must take her dietary supplements. When you hand her the first tablet and a glass of water or juice, explain to her what these supplements are and how they will benefit her: "These are your vitamins, Mom. I've noticed a real improvement in your health since you've been taking them. Now, here's the first one: it's easy to swallow. Then take sip of juice and swallow everything." Give her each tablet with the same thorough explanation, if it's necessary. Remember that tomorrow you'll go through the same routine all over again.

If your mom can't swallow her pills, try crushing them and mixing them with something tasty, like chocolate frosting, applesauce, jam, or even ranch dressing. You might want to taste each one of her supplements to find food or drink that would disguise a foul-tasting pill. Some medications, such as B complex vitamins, can't be disguised no matter what you do, although some sublingual vitamin B does come in a fruit flavor.

Be honest with her when you present her with a teaspoon of the unusual mixture: Say, "Mom, I've mixed your pill with some jelly. It still tastes a little weird, but it's not too bad." If you continue to have problems even with crushed pills, ask your pharmacist for liquid versions. Many painkillers, cold remedies, and multivitamins are available in liquid form.

(*See also:* Coaching; Honesty; Medication; Routines)

■ ■ ■ ■ ■ ■ ■
Privacy

One common anxiety among Alzheimer's folks is the loss of self-determination. By respecting his private space, you will help your father to maintain the feeling of control over his life and his space. Even if he's bedridden, you will want to continue to knock before entering his room.

Your father lives in your spare bedroom now. He's surrounded by his personal belongings and you have a sign on his door with either his name or "Dad" on it, whichever he prefers. You respect his privacy and treat his room as his own domain, always knocking before entering, even if you must leave his door ajar so you can keep an eye on him.

Knock, knock: "Excuse me, Dad, may I come in? I would like to make your bed. Is now a good time?"

Knock, knock: "Good morning, Dad. May I come in so I can help you get dressed? Then we'll eat breakfast."

Knock, knock. "Excuse me, Dad, may I come in?"

"No!"

"Oh, I'm sorry, I didn't realize you were busy. I'll come back later. Will ten minutes be good?"

"Okay."

(*See also:* Dignity; Environment; Independence)

P

■ ■ ■ ■ ■ ■ ■ ■

Projects

You and your grandmother can create art out of anything, from string and fabric to old toothbrushes. You paste things onto cardboard, mount them in boxes, or make freestanding sculptures. Remember, there are no rules on what is or isn't art! Your grandmother may not be able to start or stay with a project if she's on her own, in which case you can take advantage of the situation and work with her, adding some fun to your own day.

IDEAS

> Cardboard milk cartons make wonderful "shrines." You can cut out the front panel or divide it into two folding-door panels and spray paint it gold, silver, or any color of your choice. Then you can place an arrangement of little items you've collected inside your shrine, such as, pinecones, tiny thumb-sized dolls, broken brooches, pebbles, or leaves. You can paint them or leave them in their natural state. What you put in the shrine is entirely up to you.

> Flowerpots, baskets, or picture frames all make good starts for art pieces. You can decorate them with ribbons and odd buttons, paint them, decoupage them with magazine pictures, or cover them with pieces of differently shaped pasta and spray paint.

> Found objects can become "sculptures" by using materials from nature like leaves, twigs, cones, and nuts. Also wood scraps, hardware, broken tools, nuts, bolts, old kitchen tools, old flatware, broken dishes, pottery shards, pieces of tile, party favors, small toys, watch parts, and old jewelry can be used to good effect. You can mount your objects with white glue, contact cement, or Liquid Nails, or set them in tile-setting cement.

P

COLLAGES   You might have discovered how to make collages by accident. You ran out of gift-wrap while wrapping presents, so you used plain tissue paper and then cut out colorful pictures from old magazines and pasted them all over the tissue. Your wrapping paper was the hit of the party. You had so much fun that you decided to try it again, this time on posterboard. Since then you've collected a big box full of all sorts of images for your collages.

Because your cousin Tilda loves animals, you collect old *National Geographic* magazines and nature calendars for her. To help Tilda make a no-fail collage, you start by covering the posterboard with colored paper, construction paper, or calendar pictures. Tilda can cut out pictures, using safety scissors if necessary, but she may have trouble handling the glue stick, so help her paste the cutouts where she places them. You'll get the best results if you avoid cutting straight edges and have the pictures overlap each other. Here are some ideas:

> A big tree collage composed of images from a nature calendar. You can use tiny cutout pictures of birds and paste them all over the "branches" of the collage trees.

> A collage of desserts from food or home magazines.

> A glamour collage: Start with a large picture of a woman's face and surround her with lots of tiny overlapping cutouts, so that at a distance they look like cascading hair.

As you gain creative confidence, you can make a collage of images of your family.

CRAFTS   Your grandmother often relaxed with her knitting or crochet projects when you were a kid. Recently, you found her old knitting needles and some yarns. You eagerly brought them to her, but she only fiddled with them for a while and then set them aside, seemingly having forgotten what to do with them.

Remembering how much she used to enjoy creating something, you searched for something more appropriate. You found books on crafts projects and bought all the supplies you needed: felt squares, foam balls, glue, and safe scissors. You set up everything in front of her with great expectations, but again she just stared at the pile of art supplies. Nothing you said seemed to inspire her. You said, "Grandma, see what I got for you? You can make a lovely gift . . . Cut this out . . . now this . . . fold this and glue this on . . ." and so on.

But she replied tartly, "Well, why don't you make it, if it's supposed to be so lovely?" Aha! You decided to participate. You pulled up a chair and started working on the project with her. You followed the directions closely. Halfway through, you became totally confused. Your project looked nothing like the picture in the directions. So you said, "Grandma, this doesn't look right. What do you think we should do with it now?"

At that point, you felt that you'd reached a crossroads: either scrap the whole thing or go hog wild with what you had already created. You grabbed the first thing in front of you, cut it up, and glued it on. You threw in some glitter and pieces of yarn or ribbon. After a while your grandmother joined in. It was just too irresistible.

Whatever your end result looked like, you both had a great time and you discovered the secret to success: working together. It also helped to remember there are no rules when it comes to creativity and to have no expectations of perfect results. The most important thing is to have fun. Together!

P

FIDDLE BOXES Your dad likes to keep things organized. He helps you sort the mail and painstakingly stacks magazines by titles and dates. These tasks have been successful diversions for him. You can expand on this idea by creating "fiddle boxes."

Use an assortment of old cartons or shoeboxes and load them with interesting items that lend themselves to categorizing, sorting, or counting. One box can be stocked with screws, nails, washers, and other hardware trinkets. Another can hold a collection of odd buttons. Fiddle boxes can hold fabric scraps, cookie cutters, old postcards, old jewelry, or other small items.

Keep fiddle boxes close at hand as diversions for your father when he becomes restless. Say something like this: "Dad, I really could use some help. I found this box. Look at it, it's a godawful mess. I'm just too busy right now to clean it up. Could you spare a few minutes to help me out? Who knows what interesting stuff you'll find in all this mess."

It's important that you treat these fiddle boxes as serious projects and that you're careful not to let on to him that you've created them especially as diversions for him. After he has "helped" you, you'll want to spend a few moments admiring his handiwork and be sure to thank him for his hard work.

JIGSAW PUZZLES

Years ago your wife was a whiz with those thousand-piece puzzles that would take several days to finish, but now she has trouble coping with puzzles that have only fifty pieces. You'd like to buy her jigsaw puzzles with just a few pieces, but those are usually designed for children and may feel too juvenile for her. If that's the case, consider making your own puzzles. The number of pieces should be determined by her ability; you can start with a puzzle with only five or ten big pieces, whatever you think she can handle without stress.

How to Construct Puzzles

Supplies: Foam core (a board made from two pieces of posterboard with a core made of Styrofoam), spray adhesive, a size 11 X-Acto knife, and pages from a calendar, a full-page image from a magazine, or an 8½ x 11-inch color copy of a family picture.

Have your wife select the image. Spray the back of the picture with spray adhesive and paste it on a piece of foam core that is the same size as the picture. Let it dry for a few minutes and then cut it with the X-Acto knife into no more than ten puzzle pieces. Don't worry about cutting intricate tabs or shapes; stay with uncomplicated curves.

PAINTING

Someone suggested that you try getting your dad to paint as a form of therapy. Who? Your father? The man who always thought that artists were a bunch of weirdoes? But you need something entertaining for him to do and you know he likes to do things with his hands, so why not give painting a try?

P

As with any new activity that you introduce to your father, you join in with him. You're a novice at this art stuff too, so it will be a new adventure for both of you.

You're going to experiment and mess around, so you don't want to buy expensive canvases or watercolor paper that imply expectations of "serious" work.

Instead go to your local frame shop for mat board and foam core remnants or to a variety store for posterboard. Visit your local builders' supply store or hobby shop for foam brushes, ½ inch to 3 inches wide. Lastly, buy a few bottles of water-based poster paints.

Protect your table by covering it with newsprint, butcher paper, or a drop cloth. Lay out a single piece of posterboard or a piece of mat board so that you can both work together on one painting. Most importantly, don't take this seriously! Use wide brushes to keep yourself from getting stuck on details, and remember that abstract painting is perfectly acceptable! The point of this project is to have fun, not to produce a replica of a Rembrandt masterpiece. What makes this a wonderful activity is the process of creating and experimenting together. You may not be making serious art, but you're guaranteed to make serious fun.

Wetting down the board gives the effect of watercolor and will aid in getting your colors to flow together. Dip your brush in a bright color and make a large stroke across the entire surface. Invite your dad to dip his brush into a different color and make his own sweeping stroke. Repeat this a few times and pretty soon you'll have either a mud-colored mess or an interesting "abstract" painting.

Say, "Not bad! Look at these colors and shapes. I didn't know we were such good artists, did you? Let's paint another one. Or would you like to paint on your own?" Your father is likely to need several joint sessions with you before he feels secure enough to work by himself.

SCRAPBOOKS   Your aunt Bernice is especially fond of animals and you keep a scrapbook for her in which she collects pictures cut from nature and pet magazines. Every so often you'll both sit down and look for new images. You might say, "Bernice, you said you'd like to work on your animal book. Would you mind if I helped you?"

Bernice likes to arrange her pictures. You help her write down on each page certain classifications, such as species, home countries, color, or size. You also make sure that she has a wide variety of pictures to sort through. You'll find that Bernice will become totally engrossed in these projects as long as you treat them seriously.

———————————————

Suppose your friend Ray has a passion for sports cars. For years, he collected and piled up stacks of automobile magazines in his garage. Since you've encouraged him to keep a scrapbook of his very favorites, you've found that he'll spend time happily contemplating pictures of car designs.

You can collect images of just about anything to make a scrapbook, from babies to furniture, from flowers to recipes.

(*See also*: Activities; Choices; Coaching; Dignity; Empathy; Outings; Personal Space)

P

Projects

Q

■ ■ ■ ■ ■ ■ ■ ■
Questions

Your communication with your grandmother has improved immensely since you've been following our ideas. Still, you often find yourself in a bind when you ask her questions and don't get the responses you were expecting. Try asking questions in a way that doesn't trigger immediate resistance from her. Learn how to phrase your questions so you'll get the response you desire. Instead of saying, "Do you want to take your vitamins?" (to which you are likely to get a resounding: "No!"), try the following approach: "Before you eat your eggs, let me give you vitamins. Here, take this one first. It's the one that's good for your heart. Here you are, open up your mouth wide. (Open your own mouth wide and she'll likely mimic you.) There you are! You did it! Thank you. Now you're ready for your eggs."

Your grandmother may not remember from one day to the next what you're talking about, so preface your questions with a short recap like this: "Yesterday we bought these new pads for you to wear at night. Then, if you have a small accident, you won't have to worry about it. You thought it was a good idea. You can put one on now, before you put on your pajamas. That sounds like a good plan, doesn't it?"

Be careful to ask the type of questions that don't need more than yes and no answers. They are great when you want Grandma to participate in a casual chat, but if you need her to do something, ask your question in a way that predicts the answer. If you ask, "Do you want to take a bath?" you're most likely to get a firm "No!" So, try using a more subtle approach.

Say, "Grandma, I have something to show you. Here, let me help you out of the chair. There! Now we're going down this way.

You and I went to the store yesterday and we bought a fluffy green towel. You made me promise you that you could use it today after your bath. See, now doesn't that towel feel soft?"

You'll want to phrase your questions in such a way that the natural answer will be what you want to hear. Stop and just think about this for a moment. If you say, "You don't want to do this, do you?" saying no would be the natural response. But if you say, "You want to do this, don't you?" you will be more likely get a yes. Also, if you nod your head at the same time that you ask the question, you'll elicit a positive response most of the time.

Remember that any question that presses on your grandmother's memory may upset her, so you want to be very careful with anything having to do with recall. Drop phrases like, "Do you remember?" "Don't you remember?" and "Have you forgotten?" from your vocabulary.

If you do ask a question that puts your grandma's memory on the spot, questions such as, "Do you remember how many kids Aunt Emma had?" you'll probably get a response of "No" simply because she won't be sure what you're talking about.

Grandma may recall the information you want if you preface your question with a recap or overview. For example, you could say, "I was thinking about your sister Emma. She had several kids and I've been trying to remember all of them. I remember Jim, Mike, and Sally. But I don't remember the little ones, do you?"

If she does remember more of the children, she's doing better than you at that moment. Since you've already told her that you've forgotten the rest, if she answers no, you can laugh at the two of you for having a bad memory.

It'll take some practice to get into the habit of detailed explanations, but after a while it'll become second nature to you. Your grandmother will feel less stress, and you'll sometimes get appropriate responses, which might surprise you.

(*See also:* Choices; Coaching; Communication; Listening; Normal; Validation)

Q

R

■ ■ ■ ■ ■ ■ ■ ■
Reactions

The one word that can create the most resistance between you and your mother is "No!" Even in the mildest crisis, you'll find that using that word to stop a behavior succeeds only in causing more confusion for her. At that moment, the meaning of the word often doesn't register with her; she hears only the strident tone of your voice. It doesn't stop her from doing what she's doing, it merely agitates or startles her. Instead of reacting by saying "No!" try gently, but quickly, to interrupt what she's doing in order to defuse the situation.

Suppose your mom's standing at the kitchen counter putting the finishing touches on the dinner salad. She reaches into the refrigerator and pulls out a carton of chocolate soy milk and starts to pour it, thinking it's salad dressing. Your instinct is to yell "No!" but you resist and quickly go to her. If you reach her in time, you can discreetly stop her from pouring the soy milk by putting your hand under the carton as you say, "Oops, Mom, I think you found the wrong bottle. You told me you wanted to use ranch dressing tonight. It's in that white bottle in the back of the fridge. Do you see it?"

If you don't get there in time, try using a diversion with her while you try to salvage your salad: Say, "Do you have any more energy left, Mom? You've been working so hard, but I sure could use your help setting the table. I'll be glad to finish the salad."

Try to avoid using a "No!" reaction, even when the situation is more serious. Imagine your mother has placed a potholder on top of a burner in the mistaken belief that it's a teakettle. She's about to turn on the fire. You envision your house going up in flames, so your instincts are to scream "No!" at her. Instead, take a breath as you dash to her side and quickly retrieve the potholder. Put your arms around her and take another deep breath while you say as calmly as

R

you can, "What a good idea; I could use a cup of tea right now. Do you want to fill the kettle? What flavor tea should we have?"

This incident, by the way, is a warning to pay attention to kitchen safety. You might want to take the knobs off the stove so this won't happen again.

As soon as you think you have things under control, something always happens that catches you so off guard that it's all you can do to not react. For example, imagine your mother's waiting in the car while you go to post a letter. In the two minutes you're gone, she somehow manages to remove her blouse. This wouldn't be so bad except for the fact that she's not wearing anything else underneath.

The parking lot is crowded with people and your mother's sitting half naked in full view. You're mortified and want to scream at her. You want to disown her or put her in a nursing home first thing in the morning.

Instead, take at least two deep breaths so you can get into the car with your mom and calmly open the window to cool her off and help her put on her blouse: Say to her, "It sure got hot, didn't it? I'll open this window and then I'll help you put your blouse back on. I think we should find a place to have a glass of cool lemonade. Would you like that?"

Your mom doesn't mean to upset you. In her confusion, she may not be able to think past her most immediate concern, which in this case is to cool off. She probably isn't aware that she's in the car. If you scold her, she'd only become embarrassed about something that has already happened and cannot be changed. Furthermore, because of her memory problems, it's likely she wouldn't be able to connect your reaction to the act of removing her blouse in public.

R

Imagine that one day you hear a buzzing noise coming from the garage, and you realize that your father is no longer sitting in his easy chair. You dash out to the garage, and there your dad is at your workbench with your portable saw and a very small piece of wood. A sure recipe for disaster! He's about to start cutting when you enter.

Your instinct might be to scream at him to stop, but in that moment you realize that your outburst could startle him and cause him to cut himself. Hard as it might be, you've learned to hold back your immediate reactions and stay relatively calm.

You quickly go to his side and say, "Dad, may I interrupt you? I would like very much to watch you. You are so knowledgeable and I always learn so much when I watch you. But what do you say we eat first? Lunch is ready and you look hungry. Then, later this afternoon, we can look at your plans together."

In this manner you will have avoided a potential disaster with a diversion and you'll have paid him a compliment by showing him that you are interested in his projects.

(*See also:* Coaching; Communication; Dignity;
Diversions; Empathy; Normal; Personal Space; Projects)

Reading

Your friend Maggie was once an avid reader who'd been very proud of her book collection. You've set up a special reading corner for her in your apartment with a bookshelf filled with her favorite titles. She still loves to hold a book while sitting in her big, comfy chair beside the reading lamp. She rarely gets beyond the first page, but she's still happy as a clam. The two of you can spend hours sharing your quiet reading time as you read your book and she "reads" hers.

There are other times when you'll want to enhance your shared experience by reading out loud to her. Anything can be interesting to her when you read it with enthusiasm. Try reading a "good news" item in the daily paper, though upbeat articles can be scarce and hard to find. Or you might read a cookbook out loud and fantasize about eating a huge dinner with several courses, fine wines, and rich desserts and then be able to laugh about not having gained an ounce. *Gourmet*, *Bon Appetit*, and *Saveur* magazines have especially delectable descriptions of meals.

If Maggie has a special interest in a specific subject, such as archaeology or history, then consider taking a trip to the local library in order to find books on the subject for her. She'll enjoy discovering them and it'll be a pleasure for her to hear them read aloud. When the two of you visit a library, if she shows a special interest in a specific book, you can check it out to share later.

(*See also:* Comprehension; Discussions; Outings)

■ ■ ■ ■ ■ ■ ■ ■
Reality

Your wife rarely remembers in the usual sense of the word. What often happens is that she relives rather than remembers her past experiences. The distinction between these two is very important. She is completely in the reality of a particular memory, as if it were happening all over again. You can increase the chances of successful communication with her if you try to go into her reality with her. Take each moment for what it is at that particular time. Your wife seems to exist more and more in her memories, but then, who can blame her? After all, the present can be so confusing. It's also important to remember that Alzheimer's disease specifically destroys the brain cells that govern short-term memory.

The two of you have had such a close relationship that it never crossed your mind that things could ever be different. Now you realize that although she looks and sounds like your wife, the person you knew is no longer living inside your wife's body. You keep searching for her and feel sad and angry that she's no longer there. You think that if only you could remind her of who she is, then surely she'd snap out of it. You want to shake her and see the "real" person emerge from that familiar body.

Many of us have the mistaken assumption that if we insist on reminding the Alzheimer's person that her reality is wrong, crazy, or misguided, then she'll remember and everything will be fine again, the way it once was. But it will never be the way it used to be. The best thing you can do now is to get to know and accept the new person that she has become.

Sometimes she can't remember things that just happened, yet often she can relive an event from thirty, even sixty, years ago. Your wife might say to you, "Mother's making lunch and I have to go home

R

right now or she'll be mad at me." When she does that, she's reliving a moment in time when she was a child. Try to refrain from forcing the reality of the moment on her with remarks like, "You live here! In this house! With me! And your mother died a long time ago!"

Knowing that this flashback feels totally real to her, join her in the relived experience. Put your arm around her and say, "Your mother called and said she'll be here later, so she wants us to go ahead and eat lunch without waiting for her." This seems to satisfy her at the moment, and by the time you've finished lunch, she will have forgotten all about it. Remember that when you use this kind of response, you're respecting her thoughts and feelings at that moment and your remark is, in fact, her truth, because it's based in her reality.

Suppose you're cooking dinner when your father comes stomping into the kitchen wearing big rubber boots and a rain slicker. He's furious that his friend Larry is late: "Where the heck is that guy? He knows we need to get out to the lake by dusk. Larry's never on time for anything. I don't know why I bother . . ."

Dad and Larry were best buddies as teenagers and fishing was one of their shared passions. There's no point in arguing with him that this is "here and now" and that he's eighty something and Larry died twenty years ago. At this particular time your dad's eighteen years old again. What would calm him down at this moment?

Try using a loving lie followed by a diversion. Say something like this:

"Larry called and said he'll meet you when we finish eating. Let me hang up your raincoat until you're ready to go. It's too uncomfortable to wear that at the table, isn't it? By the way Dad, you were going to tell me about that weird tool we saw yesterday at the hardware store. You said it was some kind of saw; I'll try to describe it for you . . ."

Soon he will have forgotten all about the fishing trip with his long-gone friend.

(*See also:* Acceptance; Empathy; Loving Lies; Normal; Validation)

Reality

■ ■ ■ ■ ■ ■ ■ ■
Recording Memories

There might be times when you wish that you had a camera perma-nently aimed at your husband. Only then could you capture some pre-cious moment when he comes out with a funny-sweet remark that might lose some of its charm if you tried to write it down in your journal.

If you have a camcorder, once in a while set up the camera on a high surface or on a tripod and just let it run for an afternoon. It may sound uninteresting now, but later on you will probably appreciate these tapes because they will illustrate some irreplaceable memories of your real life with your husband.

There are so many events, great and small, that you'll want to pre-serve for yourself and for the family archives. They can be funny, sweet, or bizarre stories, or the occasions when your spouse gets on a roll and starts to reminisce. Even if you've heard his stories a hundred times before, try to record them for the rest of your family. They are a part of your life's history, whether or not they're true. The videos you record of your husband telling stories will be treasured in the years to come.

You can also keep a small cassette audio recorder in your purse or pocket so you can record what he has to say anytime, anywhere. You can transcribe them into your journal later.

(*See also:* Journals; Memories; Questions)

R

■ ■ ■ ■ ■ ■ ■ ■
Repetitions

Now that you've lived with your grandfather's dementia for a while, you're becoming accustomed to repeating your directions calmly as often as you think it is necessary. Suppose your grandfather's trying to put on his shoes. He can't quite figure out how to position his foot, so you guide it into the first shoe, while you explain to him, "We'll put the shoe here in front of you, then you can slide your toes inside and then the rest of your foot. Just like that! You've got it!"

Then you repeat the exact same directions with the second shoe. This repetition used to be maddening, but now you're accustomed to coaching him through dressing, eating, bathing, walking, and any other actions that may bewilder him. Your cheerful attitude keeps him feeling cooperative and secure. After particularly confusing times when it's clear to you that he's trying really hard, it's so natural for you to respond to him with a big hug.

Your uncle Ted tells a handful of old stories so often that you know them all by heart, yet he has trouble remembering the simplest things like where the bathroom is or how to hold a fork. It's helpful to put up signs to direct him to the bathroom, and you can place the fork in his hand as you direct it gently to his mouth.

You patiently talk him through the motions: "Here's your fork, uncle Ted. You hold it in this hand, then pick up a bite of food, and then you bring it to your mouth." Hopefully, he will remember this by the next bite, but chances are good that you'll have to repeat these directions several times during the meal. It's hard not to become impatient with him with such continuous repetition, and a few times you've slipped and blurted out, "But I just showed you how to do that!"

But when you did that, unfortunately, you just reminded him of his problem. It's likely that your uncle responded to you with increased confusion. You need to help him calm down again. You can offer to warm his food, add some more gravy, or ask him if he wants a pickle. Any of these diversions may get him refocused and give you a chance to start over again.

(See also: Coaching; Communication; Questions)

Respite

Taking care of a person with Alzheimer's is a major undertaking that should be shared, and you have the right to insist that other family members pitch in. Arrange for your siblings or other family members to stay with your mother at your house for long weekends or have your mother spend time at their homes so that you can take a break. This will not only give you the time off you deserve, it will also give them the chance to participate in caring for her, so they can see for themselves how she's really doing.

You and your mom get along well from day to day. You've set up a personal space for her, which keeps her happily occupied while giving you a little time for yourself. You've gotten pretty good at communicating with her, even as she's losing her speech. You've put up signs all over the house to help her function on her own. Everything seems fine, but there are still times when you feel trapped by your situation and you feel guilty and ashamed that you feel that way. You need some relief!

In addition to being the sole caregiver for your mom, you also may have a full-time job. This probably leaves you with little or no private time. Take advantage of all the support that is available to you. The Alzheimer's Association holds support group meetings in most communities, and local government agencies on aging can direct you to programs that can provide some respite for both you and your mother.

With any luck, your city has an adult day-care center where your mother can spend a few hours several days a week. You can also ask your local Alzheimer's Association or senior center to help you make contact with one or two other families in order to create a share care group. Sharing outings with such a group is more fun and easier on individual caregivers. Also, you can take turns caring for all your elders for a day.

Although you may find it hard work looking after more than one elder at a time, it'll be well worth it. When it's your turn to take a day off, you can blissfully enjoy it, knowing that your mother is in a safe and loving environment where she's being cared for by people who are familiar to her.

Your share care group can also take turns relieving each other in the evenings. You're all entitled to a periodic night out, to have dinner with friends, or to go to the theater or a movie, or to get a massage.

When you feel refreshed and invigorated, you can approach your caregiving tasks with new energy. Your mother will reflect how you feel by her mood and behavior.

(*See also:* Day Care; Family; Home Help; Share Care; Support Groups)

R

■ ■ ■ ■ ■ ■ ■ ■

Restaurants

Going out to eat is a special event for your sister. She'll look intently at the menu, even though it's often upside-down. She remembers the concept of reading, but she's not exactly sure how to do it anymore. Let her hold the menu any way she wants, while you read out loud from your own menu. You can point out her favorite dish: "Look Sis, they have your favorite dish. Would you like to have that today, or would you like to try something new?"

No matter how she responds, you can order something you know she'll be able to eat without too many difficulties, and when it comes to your table you present it to her with a big smile. Say, "Here it is, just what you ordered. It sure looks delicious." She may become confused if there are too many different kinds of foods on her plate, or if she's given too many utensils at one time.

Ask the waiter to bring an extra plate so you can separate fork food from finger food and serve her one kind at a time. Give her one utensil, either a fork or spoon, whichever is appropriate for the dish. It's important for her dignity that she continues to use the appropriate utensils for as long as she can. She may not be able to handle a knife efficiently or safely, so you can either choose something that doesn't need cutting or you can cut it up for her in advance.

R

Suppose your sister wants a sandwich, but her hands have forgotten how to hold it. You can either cut it up so that she can eat it with a fork, or ask the waiter to bring the contents of her sandwich without the bread, so she can eat it with a fork.

Try to allow yourself plenty of time for lunch and let your sister set the pace. You may want to frequent cafeterias or buffet restaurants where the waiters aren't dependent on tips and turnover. That way you can take your time and linger over your meal. It's important, however, to eat at restaurants occasionally because the experience can make your sister feel elegant and special. Consider going to restaurants during off-hours, either before or after the crowds.

On your ride home, you can talk to her about how nice the meal was and she can help you make plans for a return visit. You can reiterate with her what you had both enjoyed. Also, you can compare and discuss the ingredients of the meals you ate. Talking about your meals in such minute detail helps her stay with the immediate memory. Be sure to repeat several times how much you enjoyed sharing this experience with her. Restaurants make great conversation topics, because food is something we can all discuss, and we usually have strong opinions and likes and dislikes.

(*See also:* Coaching; Crowds; Dignity; Eating; Outings)

■ ■ ■ ■ ■ ■ ■ ■
Routines

Routines are often very important to folks with dementia. A routine gives them a sense of security since they know when it's time to bathe, put on shoes, or eat. Your mother grew up in a family that followed strict routines. Even though she has dementia, she still likes to do things in a certain way and at certain times. She's reassured by the familiarity of habit.

She'll set the table for you, always laying out the silverware just so, the napkins absolutely perpendicular, and her chair always facing in a particular direction at the table. Almost every day she'll insist that dinner should be on time. Your personal lifestyle is usually much more relaxed, so it can be annoying when she becomes so controlling and inflexible.

But you're learning to adjust to life by the clock, much to your mom's relief. When she is happy, life is a lot easier for the both of you. You have learned to take advantage of her near-obsessive thinking by posting a couple of big signs noting her weekly bath time. What used to be a major battle has become relatively easy now, because if she resists bathing, you can simply point to the sign in the bathroom. Say to her, "Well, let's see, here it says: Bath time—Wednesday at 2 P.M. Well, today is Wednesday and my watch says two o'clock. How about yours? I'll be glad to give you a hand. I'll start the water while you choose the soap."

R

You can keep signs in the bathroom that say: "Mom's Soap," "Mom's Towel," "Mom's Bath Time: Wednesdays." This will help maintain your bath routines.

(*See also:* Bathroom; Bath Time; Coaching; Dental Health; Dressing; Eating)

R

S

■ ■ ■ ■ ■ ■ ■ ■

Safe Return

Sponsored by the Alzheimer's Association, the Safe Return program assists in the safe and timely return of a person with Alzheimer's disease or dementia who wanders. It works very simply: When you register, for a modest fee, you are supplied with an identification bracelet or necklace engraved with

Memory Impaired
To help (Person's Name) call (800) 572-1122,
ID #_____

If your Alzheimer's person wanders off, anyone who encounters him or her can call the hotline twenty-four hours a day. The hotline will then contact you with the person's location. In a similar manner, you can call the hotline to alert them when your Alzheimer's person has gone missing. The program maintains a national database that includes important emergency contact information and photographs to help unite lost individuals with their caregivers, no matter where they may wander. Contact Safe Return at (888) 572-8566, or call the Alzheimer's Association at (888) 572-3900.

(*See also*: Identification; Neighborhood Flyer; Wandering)

■ ■ ■ ■ ■ ■ ■ ■

Sexuality

Alzheimer's disease will occasionally cause a person to express long-repressed antisocial behavior, and there are times when an Alzheimer's person will exhibit inappropriate sexual behavior. If this issue poses a problem for you, discuss it with a psychologist.

We all need to feel we are loved. An Alzheimer's person is no exception. Nursing homes frequently witness blossoming romances between residents. Usually, it's limited to holding hands and snuggling like teenagers.

Your mother has been going to the monthly socials at the senior center. When you drop her off you know that she's in a safe place, and you can treat yourself to a much-needed few hours of respite. She still loves dancing to the oldies. Lately, she's had one steady dance partner and they have such a good time that you invite him to have dinner at your house. He lives alone and reciprocates. Before long, they're seeing each other frequently. You drive your mom to his place and occasionally you drop them off at a restaurant or movie theater.

One day you arrive early to pick up your mother and you find the two of them locked in a passionate embrace. You're shocked. It had never occurred to you that there could be anything physical between them. Sure, you'd read many articles about sex in old age, but you never thought of your mother in those terms. To tell the truth, you've never thought of her as a sexual being, even when she was a young woman. Few of us think of our parents that way.

When you've had a chance to calm down, you might realize just how lucky your mother is. This charming man is obviously fond of her and accepts her, dementia and all, so try to do all you can to support their relationship. From now on be extra careful to arrive on time. Furthermore, when he visits at your home, do what you can to respect their privacy when he visits her in her room.

Your mom's beau often acts as an interpreter for her with you and others from the outside world. He is one person who truly knows what you're dealing with and with whom you can discuss difficult situations. In fact, he could become your strongest ally.

Your father and mother have both been living with you because of your mom's severe dementia. They still have an active sex life. Suppose one evening you hear a bloodcurdling scream coming from their bedroom. It's your mother's voice, and she is screaming, "Don't touch me! Get this man out of my room! Who are you? Get away from me!" And your father comes flying out of the room, half-naked and near tears. He tells you, "Your mother threw the phone at me. She doesn't know who I am. Oh God, what am I gonna do?"

You quickly give your father a hug and dash to your mother's side to calm her down. But she's fine. She has no memory of the event; she's oblivious to what has just happened.

You've never had to talk to your dad about their private life before, but now you've been thrown right in the middle of it. Invite him to talk about his feelings and let him know that you understand his distress. If he's comfortable with the idea, suggest to him that he limit himself to affectionate stroking, hugging, holding, and touching, so your mother might be less likely to freak out. Encourage him to talk to about this to his support group and offer to accompany him for emotional support, because he might be very uncomfortable discussing his private life with a group. After all, his generation believed in keeping one's feelings private, especially for men.

DELICATE SITUATIONS
It's a beautiful morning. You have a wonderful day planned, so you're feeling great when you go to wake up your mother. You knock on her door and she doesn't answer, which isn't unusual, so you walk in. But you stop dead in your tracks when you realize that your mom is contentedly playing with herself. She doesn't see you, so you make a fast exit. Objectively, you know that masturbation is a perfectly natural, normal, human activity, but *your mother*? You also know that your mom would positively die of embarrassment if she knew that you'd seen her.

For a moment you're gasping for air. So take a deep breath and ask yourself, "How am I going to deal with this?" Then take another deep breath and retreat to the kitchen to calm down. There really isn't anything you can do about it, other than to make sure that from this day on you won't be so quick to enter her room.

You may learn to look at your mother with different eyes now, realizing that she's still a woman with normal physical urges, just as you are.

S

Your uncle Dan's been fondling himself lately. When this occurs at home, you gently guide him to his room while speaking to him in a calm and normal tone of voice. Say something like, "Dan, how about spending a little private time in your room?"

If it happens in public, take a deep breath before you quietly say to him, "Dan, I think you should wait until we get home." If he doesn't relate to what you're saying, try to distract him with a forceful remark like, "Dan, your shoe is untied." Or "Oh look Dan, there's our coffee shop. You wanted a cup of cappuccino. Come, let's go." Then take him by his arm and discreetly pull his hand away. Start walking with him right away to get his mind onto your new destination.

Suppose one day your father reaches for you in an intimate way and calls you by your mother's name. Most likely, you would be horrified, but you pull yourself together and hold him at arm's length and say, "Dad, I'd like to wait until after dinner for that hug. I appreciate it though."

He may be embarrassed if he realizes what he has done, but you can comfort him by taking his arm and saying, "You must miss Mom very much. I know it's hard for you. I love you and I'm so glad you're here with me." Then, ask him to take a break with you to enjoy some music and to chat about some of the outings you are planning to take together.

(*See also:* Dignity; Empathy; Independence; Privacy; Support Groups; Validation)

S

■ ■ ■ ■ ■ ■ ■

Share Care

Both you and your mom are going to need breaks from your daily routines as well as from each other. If you have family members living in the vicinity, ask for their assistance. Review the sections in this book on Respite and Day Care. Another option you might consider is a novel concept we've chosen to call *share care*. It's a reasonable alternative to day care and senior centers, and it doesn't have to cost you anything other than perhaps the cost of a movie or a meal.

Share care works by connecting with other caregivers in your local Alzheimer's group or senior center. Periodically, you get together in small groups, that is, two or three caregivers and their Alzheimer's people. You meet for leisurely lunches at each other's homes, go to the movies together, or go out to dinner. This can be a chance to develop social relationships for both you and your Alzheimer's person. But, most importantly, this is also a great opportunity for you to generate a reliable network of caregivers who can cover for each other in emergency situations or if one of you needs a break for an afternoon.

Please remember one ironclad rule: It may be tempting to share your woes when you are out with this group of sympathetic people, but you all need to make an agreement ahead of time that any conversations about caregiving problems should be reserved for separate telephone conversations away from your Alzheimer's people's earshot.

(*See also*: Day Care; Family; Respite; Support Groups)

■ ■ ■ ■ ■ ■ ■ ■

Signs

Most Alzheimer's people retain their ability to read short sentences or single words, even while their dementia progresses. Simple signs often help keep them oriented. Use bold and clear lettering. Wall signs are best mounted at comfortable eye level. If your grandfather tends to hunch over, hang the signs where they can be seen without him having to strain his neck. The next step is to check the lighting in your house. Signs won't help if it's too dark for him to read them.

S

CRASH! Imagine that it's four o'clock in the morning, and you are fast asleep when you're abruptly awakened by the sound of a crash coming from the living room. You fly out of bed in a panic, with visions of your granddad lying on the floor with a broken leg. You run down the hallway toward the source of the noise, flipping on the overhead lights as you go. Your grandfather is standing next to a shattered lamp with a look of extreme urgency on his face. So you guide him quickly into the bathroom, just in time.

The next day you resolve to make your grandfather's life (and yours) easier. If you know that he still recognizes simple words, you can mount a series of signs on the walls of your home.

Position "Bathroom" signs with arrows pointing the way in the hallway at eye level. And post a very large sign on the door of the bathroom itself. Next, put signs on your granddad's room and on the doors of the other rooms indicating the purpose of each; that is, label them "Living Room," "Kitchen," "Dining Room," and so on. Also label items that your grandfather needs to identify, such as the laundry basket and the wastebasket. Don't panic: You don't have to do all of this in one day. You can make up, add, change, or replace the signs as necessary.

You can introduce your granddad to the signs you will make over the next few days by gently guiding him to each sign and reading them out loud. After several repetitions, it's likely he'll be able to follow them on his own.

Put a "Stop! Don't Go Out This Door!" sign on the inside of all exit doors and any other doors that need to be secure.

———————————

Your aunt Betsy's vision isn't good, so she often hangs a dress back in the closet, even when it's dirty. Doing the laundry was a major chore in Betsy's youth and one did not wash a dress until it really needed it. When you try to convince her that her dress should go in the wash, she gets very upset.

When you say, "Betsy, let's wash that dress," she responds, "But it's not dirty!" If you say, "But Betsy, you've worn that same dress for the last three days in a row," she says, "Look at it: it's not dirty! There's no point in washing it; it's a waste of soap and water."

You try to reason with her and say, "I have to wash all these other things in the hamper anyway, and there's enough space left over for your dress, so we're not using any extra soap or water. Go ahead and put your dress in the hamper."

At that point, Betsy peers down into the hamper full of underwear and socks and says, "I can't put my dress in there with those dirty things!" Before she gets upset again, gently take the dress from her, being careful to keep it separate from the other laundry as long as she's watching.

Try putting a sign on the hamper: "All Dirty Clothes Go Here." If that doesn't work for Betsy, buy a two separate plastic hampers for her clothing. Mark one "Dresses Only" and the other "Other Dirty Clothes."

(*See also:* Fixations; Home Safety; Obsessive Behavior; Wandering)

■ ■ ■ ■ ■ ■ ■ ■
Singing

No one in your family had much of an ear for music, so when your mother starts to sing along with a radio station featuring "oldies but goodies," you're quite surprised. To your amazement, she recalls most of the lyrics and happily belts them out full blast and totally off-key. Try to work up the nerve to hum along. The car's a safe place for belting out old standards, on or off-key. You may sound like cats whose tails have been slammed in a door, but who cares? You're having a good time and you're sharing some good laughs.

If your mother is mostly nonverbal, encouraging the grandchildren to sing along with her can create a special connection for them all. Besides, children can accept us just the way we are and they will generously forgive our imperfections.

Your local library has music books, audiotapes, and CDs galore. And there are tapes and CDs on the market that are especially suitable for sing-alongs of oldies and goodies.

S

(*See also:* Children; Laughter; Music)

■ ■ ■ ■ ■ ■ ■
Stress

You are, or you soon will be, an expert on stress. When you are a caregiver for a person who has Alzheimer's, to some degree stress is

unavoidable, but there are also things you can do to relieve and minimize its effects on you.

Looking after your father takes a lot of your energy, so you need
to find ways to cope while keeping your own spirits up. Also, because
your dad is so dependent on you, he will often reflect your moods and
stress. Try to maintain a balance between your own needs and his.

Make time to get a massage for yourself or have an evening out
with your friends. Continue to pursue your own interests and hob-
bies. When you plan activities to do with your dad, choose some that
you'll enjoy as well. You can encourage him to help you make a wild
sculpture or to dig in the earth. Listening to soft music for relaxation
or curling up with a good book can benefit both of you. If you have a
dog or cat, you and your father can spend time together taking a dog
for walks or grooming and petting a cat. Cuddling with a warm, fuzzy
creature can be very soothing.

Consider taking a yoga or a stress-management class. And don't
forget the value of talking to others who are in the same situation.
Attending meetings of your Alzheimer's support group or visiting a
counselor or therapist could be invaluable help for maintaining your
sanity.

(*See also*: Counseling; Day Care; Pets; Respite; Share
Care; Support Groups)

■ ■ ■ ■ ■ ■ ■ ■

Sundowning

If your wife tends to become restless at the same time every afternoon, she may be *sundowning*. This term is used to describe the agitation that occurs regularly in the late afternoon for some people with
Alzheimer's or dementia. This agitation is thought to be a chemical
reaction in the brain that's triggered by the waning light at the end
of the day.

Your wife's restlessness could be sundowning or simply a reaction to her old, built-in body clock. Someone who spends a lifetime
doing a particular job with regular hours develops an internal clock
that does not necessarily turn itself off at retirement. If your wife

used to start dinner every day at four o'clock, it's natural for her to start getting anxious and fidgety at that time of day. Encourage her to help you with cooking or table-setting tasks.

———————————

Alicia has been living in a care facility for a while now. Suppose that one day the supervising nurse tells you that Alicia is sun-downing. Before you take the staff's word for it, first find out whether they have regularly scheduled afternoon activities. Many residents are simply bored and frustrated because of idleness. Boredom and frustration can cause behavior similar to sundowning. Spend an afternoon at the home, and if you suspect that her frustration is due to boredom, talk to the management about establishing some afternoon activities.

You also can suggest to the staff that they can calm Alicia with a diversion. Give them some ideas. Suggest that they tell her she can relax because it's her day off and someone else is cooking dinner today. She also may calm down if they ask her to help set the tables or to serve the water with dinner.

(*See also:* Diversions; Empathy; Kitchen; Music; Personal Space; Projects)

■ ■ ■ ■ ■ ■ ■ ■
Support Groups

As you face your daily challenges with your mother, you might begin to doubt your caregiving skills. We recommend that you seek as much outside support as you can gather. First of all, ask your family to help you look after your mother. Caring for a person with Alzheimer's is an undertaking that needs to be shared by the whole family. Seek out one of the support groups sponsored by the Alzheimer's Association, and look into respite care, day care, and share care. Consider hiring a companion for your mom to take some of the load off your shoulders. Also look into counseling for yourself so that you'll have a safe outlet for expressing your feelings as well as a source for personal guidance.

You regularly attend your local Alzheimer's Association support group meetings. Most of the time this group is a real lifesaver for you.

S

You're able to talk openly about some of your most uncomfortable feelings, such as the guilt, resentment, and fear that often trouble you. It's reassuring to be able to share your anxieties and uncertainties with the other members of the group.

However, if the meetings have turned into gripe sessions. You come away from meetings with more negative feelings than positive ones. It's important to understand that a support group loses its effectiveness if it becomes a forum used solely to complain. How can you help the group to make a turnaround?

First, bring up the subject at the next meeting. It may be difficult, but it's likely that your feelings are shared by many of the others in the group. If they are receptive, explore together how the support group members can maintain a balance between expressing their feelings and fears and helping each other find positive solutions to their particular challenges. It will help to share this book with everyone in the group.

If you find strong resistance to this discussion, then the group may not be the right one for you. You can find another Alzheimer's support group through the Alzheimer's Association. There are often several support groups in the same area, or you can start your own with people you meet at the senior center.

(*See also:* Respite; Share Care)

S

T

■ ■ ■ ■ ■ ■ ■ ■

Telephone

The telephone is such a wonderful tool, it's a wonder we ever functioned without it. This connection with the outside world is one of the hardest thing for us to give up. A person with short-term memory loss can forget the phone call she just made and call the same person back minutes later. This can cause a lot of strain on family and friends, especially when the calls are indications of confusion or stress.

Since you moved away from home, you and your mother have stayed in touch with each other with frequent telephone calls. Lately, she often sounds surprised to hear your voice, although you've always called her before going to church on Sundays.

Then, one evening you return from work and you find that your telephone answering machine has seventeen messages on it; fifteen from your mother. You listen anxiously to each message expecting a catastrophe, but she just sounds scared and confused about the answering machine itself, although she has used it confidently for years.

On a few of the messages, she's crying. Of course, you immediately call her back, out of your mind with worry. She is delighted to hear your voice. She's is also surprised when you mention the fifteen calls, and denies making them. Clearly, she has no memory of calling you at all.

You start spending some time with her in her home, long enough to satisfy yourself that she's still okay living by herself. Apparently, the persistent telephone calls are an isolated problem. She now calls you regularly, many times a day, always forgetting that she called a short time previously. Telling her this only causes her to become more agitated and insecure, which, in turn, compels her to call more frequently.

Here's one suggestion that might work for you, but it has to be handled with great sensitivity. You can order a second phone line for all other calls and keep your regular line only for your mother since she is likely to know your number. Then program your voice mail with a message especially for her. Have your message say, "Hi Mom, this is (your name). This is my answering machine, so you can leave me a message. I'm so glad you called. I always enjoy hearing from you. I hope you're having a wonderful day. I'm a little busy right now, but I'll call you back as soon as I can."

Your latest telephone bill shows a rather sizable charge for a few dozen long-distance calls to one number: your sister's answering machine. Your poor sister! And no one knows whom else your mom's been calling. She always loved to talk on the phone. Now that she's becoming increasingly confused about it, she'll sometimes answer the phone politely and then hang up on the caller immediately.

The next time you see her reach for the phone, you can gently intercept and cheerfully tell her about the wonderful conversation that she just had (even if it was yesterday's conversation). Then use one of your effective diversions. Say something like, "Mom, let's go in the kitchen and look at the fashion catalog that came in the mail this morning. Maybe we can find a new pair of walking shoes for you."

When diversions like this no longer work, consider taking stronger measures, such as keeping the phone out of sight inside a cabinet or drawer. If your mother discovers your ruse, you can unplug the phone until you're ready to use it and tell her that it's out of order. To be convincing, you may have to sound a little annoyed with the phone company. Say to her, "Things just aren't as reliable now as they were in the old days."

Let your family and friends know what the situation is, so they can call back if your mother hangs up on them or they can leave messages for you on your voice mail.

(*See also:* Diversions; Personal Space; Projects)

Telephone

■■■■■■■■
Television

Your aunt Bertha's been watching her soap opera faithfully for years, but one afternoon she becomes very agitated and is on the verge of tears. As far as you can tell, the story line is no different from the normal drama and tribulations of all the previous episodes. So you turn the sound down on the television and ask, "Bertha, what's happening? Why are you so upset?" She responds with, "She lost the baby, she lost the baby. Oh, it's terrible." So you say to her, "Bertha, she's an actress. She didn't really lose a baby. It's only make-believe."

Bertha pays no attention to you and justs keeps repeating, "But she just lost the baby, she lost the baby." There seems no way to soothe her right now. You fetch a tissue and wipe her tears. Then you realize that to calm her down you need to go into her reality with her. Tell her, "I'm really sorry about the baby. We can write her a condolence card, okay? We can go to the card store together and pick out a beautiful card, but would you like a glass of grape juice first?"

You realize that she now has trouble distinguishing between fact and fiction. From now on, you'll need to monitor her television viewing and watch any questionable material beside her. Also, you may want to avoid watching the evening news because of its graphic content.

Looking at television through your aunt's eyes, you'll find that much contemporary humor tends to be raunchy or mean-spirited, and action programs often portray violence more graphically than she may be able to handle. If Bertha really enjoys watching television, you can rent or purchase videos of special interest to her, first making sure that none of them have emotionally wrenching content.

(*See also:* Comprehension; Movies; Reality; Videos)

T

■■■■■■■■
Transitions

Suppose you've found a really good care facility for your grandmother, now that she's reached the stage in her dementia where it has become too difficult to care for her at home. It would be wise to avoid discussing her impending move too far in advance. That way you won't cause her any unnecessary anxiety.

You remember the trauma when she first came to live with you, so you're determined to do all you can to make her move to her new environment as easy and as stress free as possible. You can make arrangements with the facility to take at least several weeks to integrate your grandmother into her new home. Your goal is a gradual transition.

Two weeks before her scheduled move, make arrangements for the two of you to eat at least two or three meals at the care facility during the first week. On your way there, talk with her as if it were just another outing: "Grandma, I thought we'd try a new place for lunch today. I hear they have good food and there are some really nice people there."

Then, on the way home, say something like this to her: "I really enjoyed that lunch. The food was good, don't you think? And such nice people, especially that lady in the blue dress. She really liked you. You know, I'd like to go back again, wouldn't you?"

The second week, go to the facility every day, alternating between lunch and dinner. When you get home, continue to discuss your "new favorite place." During this week, also join your grandmother in some of the facility's activity programs. In addition, encourage her to spend more time visiting with her future roommates. At this point, introduce the idea that it would be a good place to live: "Grandma, we have to get going now, but it sure would be so nice to spend more time here, don't you think?"

Consider all the variations on this approach and then increasingly build on the idea of living there: "I'm sorry we had to leave so soon. I know you'd like to spend more time with your friends, wouldn't you? You know, they really like you and they seem sad every time you have to leave. I wonder if they might have a room there for you. Wouldn't that be great? Then you'd be close to your friends all the time. We can ask, right? Cross your fingers."

Finally, on the day before her move, be really excited: "Grandma, I have the best news for you! I just got a phone call from your favorite place and they saved one of their best rooms for you. Isn't that exciting? I told them that you'd be very happy to hear that.

We'd better jump on it before they give it to someone else. Come on, let's celebrate!"

On moving day, take her to the facility in the morning and let her mingle with her friends while you discreetly move her belongings into her room. Be sure her pictures and possessions are in place before you bring her to it. Walk her in as if it were the executive suite at a four-star hotel: "Welcome to your room, Grandma. Boy, aren't we lucky that this was available? Isn't it nice? Look at this great view (if it has one) and see how lovely your pictures look in here."

Sit down with her in her new place and have a normal, casual conversation. She'll see how comfortable you feel being there and that will help her get over any possible anxiety. Stay with her until her bedtime and try to have breakfast with her the following morning. If she gets very anxious at this point, you may have to spend the night with her.

During the next few weeks, join her for as many meals and activities as you can. You can gradually taper off to a reasonable number of visits. It's very important to let her know that you want to spend time with her there and that you'll continue to do so. It sounds like a lot of work, and it is, but taking the time now will save you the stress you would no doubt go through if your grandmother were moved in without any preparation at all.

(*See also:* Care Facilities; Empathy; Environment; Guilt)

T

U

■ ■ ■ ■ ■ ■ ■ ■
Undressing

If you have a persistent problem with your father undressing himself, especially in public, think about buying him specialty clothing that will be difficult for him to remove without your help. For example, you can buy him jumpsuits that close only in the back so he won't be able to get out of them by himself, but remember that you'll have to help him whenever he needs to use the toilet.

If you have a sewing machine, you can alter some of the garments he already wears by stitching the front of a shirt together and sewing a long zipper into the back. If you want to get elaborate, sew together the top and bottom of a sweat suit and install a very long zipper in the back to create a jumpsuit.

Suppose one day your dad walks into the dining room without a stitch of clothing on. He's as naked as the day he was born. You might gasp in shock and try not to react in disapproval, but this is unthinkable! You were raised to be modest. Your dad's nudity is so shocking that, at first, you have no idea how to handle it.

First, take a very deep breath. Then say as casually as you can, "Hi, Dad. It looks as if you couldn't decide what to wear. Come on, let's go back to your room and we'll find you a really nifty outfit for today."

Or you might say, "It's a little cold tonight. I think we should find you some clothes to put on. What would you like to wear today, your dark blue sweats? Or your beige slacks and the brown shirt we bought last week?"

The chances are good that he will cooperate with you and let you help him. There's likely to be a good reason for his nudity. He simply might have forgotten how to get dressed or how to get to the clothes in his closet. He may be too hot. If it's not a hot summer's

U

day, he might be running a temperature and this may be the only way for him to tell you that something is wrong.

If he seems well and simply doesn't want to get dressed, what's the harm of nudity at home? However, if you are not comfortable with his nudity and he absolutely refuses to get dressed in spite of your subtle suggestions, try to convince him to take a nap, and have his clothes ready for him when he wakes up. The chances are good that he'll have forgotten his reason for wanting to be nude and will get dressed willingly.

(*See also*: Coaching; Dignity; Reactions)

U

Undressing

V

■ ■ ■ ■ ■ ■ ■ ■

Validation

A conversation with a severely confused person may be sprinkled with comments that seem to make no sense because they sound completely out of context. However, he may seem to think the comments are quite appropriate to the topic. Whatever he comes up with, try as best you can to treat him with respect.

Regressions into the past experienced by a person with dementia are as intense and as real to him as anything happening in the present. All the feelings and thoughts these memories arouse are as real as any experience you might have now. It's important not to dismiss these experiences. When you acknowledge the person's feelings and thoughts you're reinforcing his or her self-esteem.

Suppose your father is a war veteran. No one really knows what kinds of nightmarish experiences he underwent while in combat. He has always refused to discuss his war experiences, shrugging questions off with this response: "What's done is done. No point in discussing it." However, in his dementia, some of his wartime fears are coming back to haunt him. For instance, he may fixate on an enemy he thinks is coming to get him and say, "They know where I am. They're coming. They're coming to get me. Oh, what am I going to do?"

You won't have any idea who "they" might be, but that doesn't matter; what he needs is comfort and reassurance that he won't be harmed by anyone. Say to him something like this: "You're safe here, Dad. I'll never let them hurt you. Besides, they don't know this address and we have a good strong lock on the door. Would you like to see it?"

To help him calm down, you may have to make some "phone calls" to "authorities" once you find out which authorities he would trust. Within his earshot, but with the phone disconnected, pick up the phone and say, "Hello, is this the FBI? I'm double-checking our security arrangements. Will you please confirm that they don't know our address? . . . Thank you so much. I feel so much better now."

After you make the "call," you can say to your father, "Yes, Dad, the FBI agent just told me that your file is secure and they are making sure that nobody knows your whereabouts except the people we want to visit us or call us. The FBI agent also said we can call him anytime we have a concern. He was awfully nice and helpful. He said you don't have anything to worry about. You are perfectly safe here with me."

After you have defused the situation, sit down with him and talk about his feelings to help him return to a sense of safety. Say, "Dad, I love you and I can see that it's very hard for you sometimes. I'm never going to let them hurt you again. You just let me know whenever I can help you, okay? I'm so glad that we're safe here."

Your father isn't just remembering these past experiences, he's reliving them in real time. It's important to recognize this difference and to realize that his fears are as fresh—and as frightening— now as they were then. Sometimes it's hard for us to understand how someone who appears to be so confused could have feelings so intense about something that happened such a long time ago. Your father has dementia, but he's still a human being with the full gamut of normal human emotions. And although the circumstances that gave rise to those emotions took place long ago, the emotions are still deeply felt in the present.

(*See also:* Acceptance; Attitude; Communication; Comprehension; Conversations; Dignity; Empathy; Listening; Loving Lies; Memories; Normal; Reality; Word Substitutions)

■ ■ ■ ■ ■ ■ ■ ■

V

Videos

Since you can't always be at your grandfather's side, videos (or DVDs) are a good alternative. He loves watching television, but you've noticed that, lately, he has difficulty distinguishing fiction from reality in many television dramas. Videos allow you to monitor what he watches to avoid unnecessary distress.

Almost any subject is available on video, from architecture to zebras. You can also find old movies on video, from Humphrey Bogart's films to Sid Caesar's television shows. Check with your local library and video stores. You might also consider videotaping his favorite television shows to play back at times better suited to his schedule.

If your grandfather was a movie fan in his youth, consider buying a collection of film classics for him. Look on the Internet for Web sites that specialize in classic movies. It may be a major investment for you, but it will be well worth it if he's happy spending hours watching his old favorites. He may not be able to follow the story line too well, especially on the small screen, but chances are good that he knows the film's plot by heart anyway. Besides, just watching his favorite actors may be pleasure enough for him. Many of the larger video rental stores have a sizable collection of the classics or are willing to order them for you.

A typical Sunday at your grandparents' house would see your grandmother and the other women in the kitchen or garden, and your grandfather and the other men in the den glued to the television set. Your granddad still enjoys watching football games, but increasingly he gets so involved in the conflict that he carries his anger into the rest of the day. As far as you can tell, his dementia is causing distortions in his perception of what he sees. He has a hard time following the game, and he even gets the commercials confused with the game.

For some time now you've been watching the games with your granddad to talk him through some of the rough spots. But you've never been a football fan and he gets upset at your ignorance. And, frankly, you can think of lots of better things to do with your time. You're looking for a way to keep both of you content. Videos might offer a solution for you. You can acquire videos of NFL highlights and NFL bloopers. Granddad can watch these videos repeatedly and, because they're familiar, the chances are good that he will not become agitated.

(*See also:* Movies; Television)

V

Videos

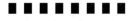

Visitors

Visits can be stressful for both the visitor and the person with dementia. Visitors have high expectations, especially if they had close relationships with the Alzheimer's person in the past. There is a good likelihood, however, that the Alzheimer's person won't even recognize the visitors. If the visitors have little prior experience with Alzheimer's, this can be very disappointing to them.

Suppose your mother's best friend from childhood, Ellen, is coming to visit from out of state for the first time in years. Lately, your mom has been quite confused and the odds are good that she won't recognize her childhood friend. You want their reunion to go well, especially for Ellen's sake. She is coming a long way with high expectations and is likely to be hurt if the visit goes badly.

Before you take Ellen in to see Mom, meet with her to help her make this a successful encounter. Explain some of the difficulties of communicating with your mother to her. Give her some examples of how to talk about their shared memories by using anecdotes and stories. Have her read the section "Memories" in this book, and emphasize the pitfalls of "Do you remember . . . ?" types of questions.

Ask Ellen to keep her tone moderate, but adult. Make it clear to her that your mother understands a lot more than appearances would suggest.

A few minutes before bringing Ellen in to see her, say to your mother, "I have a surprise for you, Mom. Your best friend, Ellen, is coming to visit us. I'm really looking forward to seeing her, and because it's been such a long time since she was last here, I wonder if we'll recognize her. She may look very different now."

Your mother doesn't handle surprise very well, so you'll have to ease her friend back into her awareness. Let Ellen know ahead of time how you intend to introduce her and ask her to wait for your cue. When you accompany her to meet your mom, say calmly and cheerfully, "Mom, I want you to meet this beautiful woman. Believe it or not, this is Ellen, your old best friend. Ellen, Mom and I are so glad you're here. Mom lives here now. I'm so lucky we have such a good time together."

V

If your mom doesn't react, keep talking to her in an adult tone of voice and gesture to Ellen to do the same. Say something like this to Ellen, "Well, Ellen, I bet Mom would like to hear how you're doing these days. Wouldn't you, Mom?"

Encourage your mother's friend to talk about her trip, her life, her pets, and other such chitchat. When you act as a go-between, your mother won't have to say a word to feel part of the conversation. Continue to assume that your mother comprehends every word. If Ellen forgets and starts talking about her as though she can't hear, you can bail her out by redirecting her questions and comments to your mom: "Mother, Ellen's asking you if your back is still bothering you. What do you say? To me, your back seems to have improved so much that you've forgotten all about it."

With your help, her friend's visit can be fulfilling and fun for all of you. Your mother may forget the event almost immediately, but it's likely that the good feelings will stay with her.

(*See also*: Communication; Conversations; Memories)

■ ■ ■ ■ ■ ■ ■ ■
Vitamins

Even if you eat a healthy diet, you still may be lacking certain crucial nutrients. To be safe, all adults should take a multiple vitamin and mineral supplement daily. The elderly need the extra protection of a multivitamin formulated especially for mature people, because with age our bodies lose the ability to absorb nutrients.

Many vitamin tablets are so large that they may be hard for your father to swallow, in which case you can purchase a liquid vitamin or you can crush them and mix them with a little jelly.

V

Antioxidants. These help to combat free radicals. Free radicals are unstable oxygen molecules, which can damage healthy cell membranes and tissue. Free radicals have been implicated in cancer, heart disease, Alzheimer's, and many other physical conditions. Antioxidants are the vitamins C, E, and beta-carotene, which are found naturally in fresh fruit and vegetables, as well as in green and black teas. (Ames 2003).

Folate (folic acid). Studies have shown that folate deficiencies aggravate brain lesions in Alzheimer's. Government research estimates that 80 percent of all Americans fall short of the federally recommended daily minimum of 400 micrograms of folic acid (Cummings and Cole 2002). The best natural sources for this vitamin are legumes, green leafy vegetables (especially spinach), citrus fruit, and whole grain products.

Vitamin E. This crucial vitamin has been found to be especially effective for Alzheimer's people. One study has shown that vitamin E taken with Aricept (donepezil) noticeably improves cognition. (Sobow and Kloszewska 2003). It may also enhance the effectiveness of other Alzheimer's drugs. A minimum of 800 IU should be taken daily. Vitamin E is available in liquid form.

Choline. Deficiency of the B vitamin choline has been shown to be a cause of Alzheimer's disease (Zeisel et al. 2003). This vitamin is crucial for muscle and nerve health. It's naturally available in foods such as liver, cauliflower, soybeans, spinach, lettuce, nuts, and eggs. Choline is also found in lecithin, which can be added to hot cereals, smoothies, or puddings.

Omega-3 fatty acids. These essential fatty acids are crucial to heart health and general cell health. Most elderly people do not get enough healthy fats in their normal diets. Omega-3s are available as a supplement made from fish or flaxseed oil, or you can add freshly ground flaxseeds and nuts to your cooking (Dixon and Ernst 2001).

V

(*See also:* Alternative Remedies; Alzheimer's Disease; Dementia; Diet and Nutrition; Medication; Pills)

W

Walking

Your wife walks very cautiously these days. She slows down and seems to feel her way with the toe of her shoe. Recently, she had her vision tested and it seems reasonably normal, so her confusion must be caused by her dementia. Because of her mobility problems you've been paying particular attention to how you yourself move about. You may have noticed that you routinely survey and register what's ahead of you as you walk. You unconsciously "memorize" the path ahead.

With that idea in mind, her behavior makes perfect sense. Your wife has trouble with abstract concepts and remembering in general, so it's no wonder she has difficulty with walking. She can't "memorize" the terrain ahead of her while she is walking.

Get into the habit of acting as your wife's eyes and memory by engaging in a descriptive commentary of the terrain as you hold her by the arm. For example, you could say, "There's a curb coming up, Sweetie. Then it's smooth for a while." As you approach street corners, you could say, "We'll go around a corner up ahead. It's a little uneven, but there are no steps."

When you come to a flight of steps inside a building, tap your toe at the edge of the first step and say, "We're going down three steps now. Here's the first one." With such descriptive commentary, you will be thinking out loud for the two of you. Before long, this behavior will become so habitual for you that you may find yourself doing it with your friends.

When you are out walking with your wife, the following instructions provide the best and safest way to hold her arm while you walk with her:

> Bend the elbow of your arm and hold her arm (which should also be bent at the elbow) close to your side.

> Clasp her hand lightly and hold her so that her elbow rests against your waist. Should she stumble, you'll have a firm and safe grip on her through the entire length of her arm, which will keep her upright and keep the risk of injury at a minimum.

> It's important not to lace your fingers together with hers. Should you need to move quickly to grab her, you would be slowed down by having to unlace your fingers. This hold will not only keep your wife stable on her feet, it will also keep the two of you side by side, making your conversations more connected and intimate. It also will help her feel equal to you.

> Avoid dragging or leading her behind you because you won't be able to see how she's moving along. Dragging and leading are also impatient maneuvers, similar to the way many of us used to drag our kids around when they walked too slowly for our adult tastes. It's inconsiderate to treat children or adults in this manner.

(*See also:* Body Language; Coaching)

■ ■ ■ ■ ■ ■ ■ ■
Wandering

Because of their tendency to wander, Alzheimer's people should *always* wear identification, either a medical alert bracelet with a contact telephone number or one issued by the Safe Return program through the Alzheimer's Association.

Suppose one morning while still in her pajamas, your mother decides to take a walk by herself. You'd gone to the bathroom for just a moment, but when you return to the living room, the front door is wide open and your mother is nowhere to be seen. A quick glance up and down the street reveals nothing. You jump into your car and

W

drive around the block, imagining the worst, of course, and then there she is, petting a miniature poodle, looking as happy as a child.

You feel so relieved and, at the same time, you want to scream at her for putting you through this trauma. Anger is a natural reaction to fear. For example, far too many of us have yelled in fear at our young children for running into street traffic after a ball.

As you climb out of the car, take a deep breath and join her while she continues to pet the dog. Take your time until you're calm again, then gently guide her back to the car, nodding a smile to any curious neighbors looking on. Your first instinct is to yell at her for scaring you so, but take deep breath instead and say, "Mom, please don't go out without me. Next time you want to go for a walk, just ask me and we'll go together. Okay?"

Say, "It sure is a beautiful day today, a great day to be outside. I really understand why you wanted to go for a walk. I'd love to come with you next time. How about this? First we'll go home and finish our breakfast, and then we can plan the rest of the day. We can go out for a walk together later today if you like. Okay?"

Now you have some decisions and preparations to make, because you know this will happen again. Is there a way to secure your home exits without feeling like a prisoner yourself?

In the city, you can enlist the help of your neighbors and alert them to the possibility of your mother's wandering. You can distribute a flyer (see Neighborhood Flyer) all around your neighborhood with her picture and a description so that people will be informed of her condition. Bring the flyer into the local shops and ask them to be on the alert for her should she wander away again.

If you live in a rural area, you may face a different set of problems. You may have to enclose your surrounding yard or garden with a secure fence. Should your mother manage to wander off in spite of all your precautions, alert your local search and rescue team right away. Your mom could easily get lost in the desert or woods and suffer from exposure or hypothermia.

Searching for your mom may be challenging. Because of her confusion, she might be very creative in her exploring; her wandering might not necessarily be logical. She may have decided to go "home," meaning back to her childhood when life was simple and safe. If she has that idea in mind, it might be natural for her to play "hide and seek," "cops and robbers," or "treasure hunt." Most likely, she won't

W

even be aware that she's "lost." As far as she's concerned, she has a definite purpose and destination.

Get her a medical alert bracelet. We recommend that you have it inscribed with "Alzheimer's." She may not have Alzheimer's disease, but it's the most recognizable term for dementia-related conditions.

Visit your local police department and hospital emergency rooms. Give them a packet of information that includes a current photo of your mother and any relevant information about her.

Your uncle Arnold immigrated to this country before you were born. He had some horrible experiences when his home country was invaded during a war. He had to go underground and barely escaped with his life. Because of his early experiences, he developed a certain anxiety whenever he was around anyone in a military style of uniform.

Nowadays, he frequently lives in an altered reality, so if he has wandered off, it's crucial that you inform the search and rescue team about his background. If he were to see police officers or sheriffs in their uniforms, the chances are good that he would remember the hide and escape methods of his youth, and he would do everything to get away from them. The search and rescue people will appreciate your information and will likely have everyone on the team wear civilian clothes to help him feel safe.

(*See also:* Identification; Conversations; Neighborhood Flyer; Safe Return)

■ ■ ■ ■ ■ ■ ■ ■
Word Games

Even if your father's verbal skills are not as sharp as they once were, there are certain things he can still recall with a little prodding from you. Proverbs, platitudes, and old sayings often stay in our memories longer than personal experiences. Games provide good stimulation when they are approached as a shared and playful experience.

Avoid competitiveness or putting anyone on the spot. Play only as long as it's fun for both of you, and remember that the most

W

important factor is the socialization that happens. Many of these games work especially well in a group, so introduce them to your share care group or try them at a family gathering.

FANTASY GAMES Imagine that your afternoon plans have been ruined by a sudden downpour. You're both disappointed, so you try a fantasy trip instead. Say something like this to your granddad, "Gee. Look at that rain, grandpa. It's too bad; we had such great plans. Our trip to the rose garden will just have to wait for a sunny day. But, I have a suggestion: how about flying to Paris for dinner at Maxim's?"

Your grandfather looks puzzled, but you continue without missing a beat: "We can spend the night at an exclusive hideaway on the Isle of Capri. Then we'll fly to Cairo for breakfast and tour the pyramids before lunch. Do you think we should bring a picnic or should we zip off to Kenya for a safari?"

If he still doesn't respond, you can elaborate and get even more playful: "Nah, I think we should climb to the top of one of the pyramids and take a rocket to Mars. I've always wanted to see the red sky of Mars. How about you? I wonder what kinds of food they serve in Martian restaurants?"

At that point, he finally might grin, having caught on to the silliness of your fantasy, so you continue, "We could take the first morning flight out and finish up by going to the opera in Sydney, Australia."

He responds, grumpily, "I don't like opera."

"Okay, then we can go to Kyoto, Japan, instead. You've always liked Japanese food and you'll love Japanese gardens."

You can continue this fantasy game indefinitely. Ask your grandfather where he'd like to go next and elaborate on each location. If you're not familiar with it, make up something fantastic and ask for his suggestions or corrections.

W

NAMING THINGS You can name car brands, states of the union, presidents, TV shows, writers, animals, countries, occupations, holidays, and so on. Or you can name vegetables, fruits, ice creams, desserts, sandwiches, and drinks. Make up a menu for a picnic, a party, or a flight to the moon. Make up weird food and drink combinations: strawberry pizza, hamburger pudding, asparagus with chocolate syrup, and so forth.

PLATITUDES This can be a fun game for just the two of you. See how long you can keep it going. You just take turns coming up with platitude or clichés. Here's an example:

"How are you doin'?"

"As well as can be, how's about you?"

"Hanging in there!"

"You sound peachy."

"Oh, it's hunky-dory."

"So you're in the pink?"

"Could be worse."

"Well, tomorrow is another day."

"One day is like another."

"Easy come, easy go."

And so on.

STORY MAKING This game can be played with a group of people or just the two of you. Go as fast you can, giving your first reactions. You'll end up with a nonsensical story, which makes this game a lot of fun. Write it down so you can share it when you've finished.

For example you could start with, "Once upon a time a . . . ?"

And your mother might respond, "crocodile."

Then you say, "He lived in a . . . ?"

And she says, "Brooklyn Bridge."

And you say, "His favorite pastime was to . . . ?"

And she says, "read."

And so on.

■ ■ ■ ■ ■ ■ ■ ■

Word Substitutions

W

Your father is losing his grasp of language and has started substituting words for those he's forgotten. If you suspect you know what he means by his substitution, use the accurate word in your response, but avoid making it sound like a correction. Most of the time it's easy to interpret what he means.

"I want more grun on my cereal."

"Would you like more milk on your cereal, Dad?"

"That's what I said!"

If you have no idea what on earth he's talking about, let your response be vague and interested enough to solicit a second remark from him. Bit by bit you'll piece it together. If he says, "Where's the green?" does he mean green shirt? Or does "green" mean something else entirely, like dog, toothbrush, or the Mozart CD? You need more to go on.

Choose a neutral response while you try to figure out what he wants. Say, "I don't recall seeing it lately, I wonder if it could be outside."

"Of course not, Stupid! I just mooed it."

Say, "I'll help you look, Dad. Was it the big one or the little one?"

"My green!" he says joyfully as he picks up a half-eaten sandwich.

He may use substitutions randomly or he may have one favorite word that he uses for anything of importance. It can be tempting to use these substitutions yourself, but try to resist. Remember that he's probably trying to find the correct word in his head, so using his substitute word may confuse or insult him.

"I want to wear the blue loyal today." (= shirt)

"You look so good in the blue shirt, Dad."

"I'm going to read my loyal now." (= book)

"I have heard it's a very good book. How do you like it?"

"I am so loyal now." (= tired or hungry?)

"I'm hungry and tired, too. I'll fix us some lunch now, and then we can take a nap afterward. Sound good to you?"

You knew he meant either hungry or tired, so with this response you have addressed both needs.

(See also: Communication; Conversations; Discussions; Questions)

W

X

■ ■ ■ ■ ■ ■ ■ ■

X-Ray

X-ray procedures can be very stressful. The labs are kept chilled and dark. Surfaces are cold and hard and the patient is required to remain absolutely still, whether lying down or standing up. This is particularly hard for an Alzheimer's person. Also, there might be additional discomfort or pain if the exam is needed to see the extent of an injury.

Suppose your aunt has a diagnosis that requires an x-ray for confirmation. Explain her dementia to the technician and request a protective lead apron. This will allow you to stay in the room while the pictures are taken. You know this is necessary to keep her calm, steady, and reassured. If she is injured, she is likely to be in pain and she's probably spooked by this alien place. You can help her to feel safer by holding her hand as you explain to her in a soothing voice why she is here, and what's likely to happen. Reassure her that it won't take too long and that you'll stay there with her. Talk to her through all the instructions.

When the technician directs her to take a deep breath and hold it, you can repeat it to her and include yourself: "We're going to take a really deep breath. Are you ready? Here we go": Breathe deep (as you breathe with her). "Now, hold it" (as you hold your breath.) Hopefully, this will work so well that you'll have to go through this exercise only once per picture. Regardless of how the session goes, thank her for cooperating and celebrate with a pleasant diversion afterward.

(*See also*: Coaching; Health; Pain)

X

Y

■ ■ ■ ■ ■ ■ ■ ■
Yeast Infections

Yeast infections are common among elderly women and, if left untreated, they can cause more serious infections. If you notice that your mother seems unusually distracted and tries to rub or scratch her groin, you'll want to examine her underwear, brief, or pad for signs of yeast, which are white or slightly green secretions. If you see this, take her to her doctor for a checkup.

(*See also:* Health)

Y

Z

■ ■ ■ ■ ■ ■ ■ ■

Zany

After living with an Alzheimer's person you've most likely become accustomed to conversations that are often totally illogical. Because Alzheimer's people live in the moment, they may go from one topic to another within the same sentence depending on what triggers their thoughts at that moment.

For example, suppose you are sitting with your father on a park bench overlooking a lake. He's enthusiastically engaged in a conversation with you. You're talking about the weather and the spring blossoms around you, when you realize from his responses that he thinks the two of you are sitting by the lake he used to visit when he was a child in a faraway place.

You do your best to join him in this altered reality, when his very next response makes it obvious that his thoughts have drifted into yet a different memory. As he watches the youngsters playing and families strolling by, each image triggers yet another reality. As hard as you try, you probably have a hard time keeping up. Such zany conversations are typical of Alzheimer's and you might as well enjoy them. There may be times when it's hard not to be amused at the inadvertently funny combinations of thoughts, but try not to laugh at them. You might even want to tape one of these precious exchanges.

(*See also:* Conversations; Reality; Validation)

Z

■ ■ ■ ■ ■ ■ ■ ■

Zippers

Zippers are a great aid in getting an Alzheimer's person dressed. They are quick and easy to use. Suppose you're having a problem because your mother likes to undress at the most inappropriate times. If you've created a few special outfits for her that zip up in the back, then her attempts to undress will be frustrated. You can sew a blouse and a pair of pants together at the waist. Sew the fronts closed and install an extralong zipper in the back. She'll still have the look of "normal" outfit, but she won't be able to remove the garment by herself.

(*See also:* Undressing)

■ ■ ■ ■ ■ ■ ■ ■

Zoos

If you and your uncle are animal lovers and you're lucky enough to have a zoo nearby, you might want to add it to your itinerary of outings. Pack a picnic lunch and go early before the crowds arrive. Find yourselves a bench or bring a couple of folding chairs. When you find an exhibit that you both like, settle down for a leisurely snack and share your observations. Social animals like apes, monkeys, and raccoons are particularly engaging. You can help your uncle express his observations by thinking out loud. "I'm watching the one down there on the side. Looks to me like she's going to be a mama soon. Or maybe she is just fat. What do you think?" If he doesn't respond, try to follow his gaze and start observing for him. "You're looking at the big male over there in the corner, aren't you? He's quite handsome, isn't he? Look at how agile he is, swinging into the branches."

Most of us dash through the entire zoo and hardly ever take the time to study individual animals. It can be a treat to concentrate on just a single group and save the rest of the creatures for another day. The other advantage is that your uncle will not be physically stressed nor overly stimulated. It's also much less confusing for the two of you later when you talk about your experiences. "What a great day we

Z

had at the zoo today. I remember that one funny little monkey who kept taking carrots from the big male and he didn't seem to notice. Would you like to go back to the zoo and visit them again soon?"

(*See also:* Outings, Pets)

Z

Resources

■■■■■■■■
Support Groups and Information

The Alzheimer's Association National Office: 919 North Michigan Avenue, Suite 1000, Chicago, IL 60611-1676. Hotline and general information: (800) 272-3900. Fax: (312) 335-1110. www.alz.org.

Most local chapters offer support groups. Call the toll-free number for further information.

ADEAR, Alzheimer's Disease Education and Referral Center: P.O. Box 8250, Silver Spring, MD 20907-8250. (800) 438-4380. www.alzheimers.org.

National Institutes of Health provide current information on all health matters. You'll find an index at www.nih.gov.

National Institute on Aging: 31 Center Drive, Bethesda, MD 20892. (301) 496-1752. www.nia.nih.gov.

National Institute of Dental and Cranial Research, NIH: (301) 496-4261.

National Eye Institute, NIH: (301) 496-5248. www. nei.nih.gov.

National Institute on Deafness and Other Communication Disorders, NIH: (800) 241-1044 or TTY at (800) 241-1055. www.nidcd.nih.gov.

Podiatric Association: (800) 366-8227. www.apma.org/foot.html.

National Hospice and Palliative Care Organization: 1901 N. Moore St., Suite 901, Arlington, VA 22209. (703) 837-1500 or (800) 658-8898 (help line). www.nhpco.org.

Ombudsman's Program, Administration on Aging: 1424 16th Street, NW, Suite 202, Wahington, DC 20036. (202) 332-2275. www.itcombudsman.org.

■■■■■■■■
Information on Long-Term Care and Alzheimer's Facilities

Senior Centers: Most towns have at least one senior center. Look for stimulating programs such as dancing, arts and crafts, and special movies.

Local Hospitals: Many hospitals have special group sessions for people with Alzheimer's and dementia. If your Alzheimer's person is able, encourage him or her to participate.

ASA, American Society on Aging: 833 Market St, Suite 511, San Francisco, CA 94103. (800) 537-9728. www.asaging.org.
    ASA hosts national conferences and offers educational programming, publications, information, and training resources for professionals in the field of aging.

NCOA, National Council on Aging: 409 Third St. SW, Washington, DC 20024. (202) 479-1200. www.ncoa.org.
    NCOA is a national voice and advocate for public policies that promote vital aging.

Safe Return (Alzheimer's Association program): (888) 572-8566 or (800) 272-3900. www.alz.org/Services/safereturn.asp.

Project Lifesaver, www.projectlifesaver.org.
    A rapid-response program that uses electronic tracking devices to locate Alzheimer's persons who've wandered off.

■ ■ ■ ■ ■ ■ ■ ■
Books

Avadian, B. 2003. *Finding the Joy in Alzheimer's: Caregivers Share the Joyful Times.* Lancaster, CA: North Star Books. www.The CareGiversVoice.com and NorthStarBooks@avradionet.com.

Goldman, C. 2003. *The Gifts of Caregiving: Stories of Hardship, Hope, and Healing.* Minneapolis, MN: Fairview Press. www.fairviewpress.org.

Mace, N. L., and P. V. Rabins. 1999. *36-Hour Day: A Family Guide to Caring for Persons with Alzheimer's Disease, Related Dementing Illnesses, and Memory Loss in Later Life.* New York: Warner Books. www.twbookmark.com.

Marcell, J. 2001. *Elder Rage, or Take My Father . . . Please! How to Survive Caring for Aging Parents.* Irvine, CA: Impressive Press. www.elderrage.com.

Salzman, C. 2002. *Psychiatric Medications for Older Adults: The Concise Guide.* New York: The Guilford Press. www.guilford.com.

Strauss, C. J. 2001. *Talking to Alzheimer's.* Oakland: New Harbinger Publications, Inc. www.newharbinger.com.

Tanzi, R. E., and A. B. Parson. 2000. *Decoding Darknes: The Search for the Genetic Causes of Alzheimer's Disease.* Cambridge, MA: Perseus Publishing. www.perseuspublishing.com.

Warner, M. 2000. *The Complete Guide to Alzheimer's-Proofing Your Home.* Jupiter, FL: Ageless Design. www.agelessdesign.com.

Weil, A. T. 1998. *Natural Health, Natural Medicine.* New York: Houghton Mifflin Co. www.drweilselfhealing.com.

Wolfe, S. M., L. D. Sasich, and R. E. Hope. 1999. *Worst Pills, Best Pills, A Consumer's Guide to Avoiding Drug-Induced Death or Illness.* New York: Pocket Books. www.worstpills.org.

■ ■ ■ ■ ■ ■ ■ ■
Alzheimer's Web Sites

www.alzforum.org.htm
  Alzheimer's research links

www.yourfamilyshealth.com/aging/
  Alzheimer's care

www.health-dictionary.com/alzheimers/
  Alzheimer's disease medical terms

www.agelessdesign.com/news-alz.htm
  Sign up for a daily e-newsletter for the latest news on Alzheimer's.

www.nutrition.org
  Information on nutrition and alternative medicines.

■ ■ ■ ■ ■ ■ ■ ■
Caregivers' Web Sites

www.ec-online.net (Elder Care Online)
  Web site and e-newsletter are excellent resources for caregivers.

www.elderrage.com
  Caregiver newsletter and links to the most comprehensive list of resources.

www.caregiving-solutions.com (Alzheimer Solutions)

www.medscape.com (Medscape Today)
  General medical information.

www.medsave.govt.ny/hot/media/2003/whims.htm (Women's Health Initiative study)

■ ■ ■ ■ ■ ■ ■ ■
Products: Call for Free Catalogs

AARP: 3557 Lafayette Rd., Indianapolis, IN 46272. (888) 687-2277. www.aarp.org

Buck & Buck Designs: Specialty clothing. 3111 27th Avenue South, Seattle, WA 98144-6502. (800) 458-0600. www.buckandbuck.com.

S&S Healthcare: Great resource for all kinds of crafts kits, games, and hobby supplies. (800) 243-9232. www.snswwide.com.

SEARS, Shop at Home: Home health care. (800) 733-7249. www.sears.com.

Wardrobe Wagon: Specialty clothing. (800) 992-2737. www.wardrobewagon.com.

■ ■ ■ ■ ■ ■ ■ ■
Identification

www.medical-id.com/: P.O. Box 50, Verbank, NY 12585. (800) 830-0546. Online links to medical identification dealers. www.medical-id.com.

■ ■ ■ ■ ■ ■ ■ ■
Legal Publications and Information

www.nolo.com

References

Aisen, P. S., K. A. Schafer, M. Grundman, E. Pfeiffer, M. Sano, K. L. Davis, M. R. Farlow, S. Jing, R. G. Thomas, and L. J. Thal. 2003. Effects of rofecoxib or naproxen vs placebo on alzheimer disease progression: A randomized controlled trial. *JAMA* 289:2819-2826.

Ames, B. N. 2003. The metabolic tune-up: Metabolic harmony and disease prevention. *Journal of Nutrition* 133:1544(S)-1548(S).

Ballard, C., J. Grace, and C. Holmes. 1998. Neuroleptic sensitivity in dementia with Lewy bodies and Alzheimer's disease. *Lancet* 351:1032-1033.

Biermann, A. 2002. Do soy isoflavones lower cholesterol, inhibit atherosclerosis, and play a role in cancer prevention? *Holistic Nurse Practitioner* 16(5):40-48.

Blaylock, R. L. 2002. *Health and Nutrition Secrets That Can Save Your Life.* Albuquerque, NM: Health Press.

Crystal, H. A., D. Dickson, P. Davies, D. Masur, E. Grober, and R. B. Lipton. 2000. The relative frequency of "dementia of unknown etiology" increases with age and is nearly 50 percent in nonagenarians. *JAMA Archives of Neurology* 57:713-719.

Cummings, J. L., and G. Cole. 2002. Alzheimer's Disease. *JAMA* 287:2335-2338.

de la Torre, J. 2004. Is Alzheimer's disease a neurodegenerative or a vascular disorder? Data, dogma, and dialectics. *The Lancet Neurology* 3(3):184-190.

Dixon, L. B., and N. D. Ernst. 2001. Choose a diet that is low in saturated fat and cholesterol and moderate in total fat: Subtle changes to a familiar message. *Journal of Nutrition* 131:510(S)-526(S).

Feinstein, J., K. M. Halprin, N. S. Penneys, J. R. Taylor, and J. Schenkman. 1973. Senile purpura. *JAMA Archive of Dermatology* 108:229-232.

Hock, C., U. Konietzko, A. Papassotiropoulos, A. Wollmer, J. Streffer, R. von Rotz, et al. 2002. Generation of antibodies specific for beta-amyloid by vaccination of patients with Alzheimer disease. *Nature Medicine* 8(11):1270-1275.

Horton, R. 2002. The hidden research paper. *JAMA* 287:2775-2778.

Johnston, C., D. R. Gress, W. S. Browner, and S. Sidney. 2000. Short-term prognosis after emergency department diagnosis of TIA. *JAMA* 284:2901-2906.

Kaplan, K. 1992. Researches find clues to cause of Alzheimer's. *The Tech: MIT.* 112(25):1, 9.

Klatte, E. T., D. W. Scharre, H. N. Nagaraja, R. A. Davis, and D. Q. Beversdorf. 2003. Combination therapy of donepezil and vitamin E in Alzheimer's disease. *Alzehimer Disease & Associated Disorders* 17(2):113–116. April/June.

Kleijnen, J., and P. Knipschild. 1992. Ginkgo biloba for cerebral insufficiency. *British Journal of Clinical Pharmacology* 34(4):352-358. Review.

Mendonça, A., F. Ribeiro, M. Guerreiro, C. Garcia, and E. Moniz. 2004. Frontotemperal mild cognitive impairment. *Journal of Alzheimer's Disease* 6(1):1-9.

Mukamal, K. J., L. H. Kuller, A. L. Fitzpatrick, W. T. Lonstreth, Jr., M. A. Mittleman, and D. S. Siscovick. 2003. Prospective study of alcoholic consumption and risk of dementia in older adults. *JAMA* 289:1405-1413.

Pratico, D. 2001. New urine test to detect Alzheimer's disease available to consumers. AlzheimerSupport.com, Alzheimer's Disease Education and Referral (ADEAR) Center. November 6, 2001.

Royce, G. 2002. WVU develops skin test to diagnose Alzheimer's. *West Virginia University News and Information Services.* September 21, 2002.

Sarrel, P. 2002. Women's Health Initiative study on HRT stopped. *Health Link,* Women's Health Initiative, Yale–New Haven Hospital. September 24, 2002.

Shaywitz, B. A., and S. E. Shaywitz. 2000. Estrogen and Alzheimer disease: Plausible theory, negative clinical trial. *JAMA* 283:1055-1056.

Shomali, M., and S. Wolfsthal. 1997. The use of anti-aging hormones. *Maryland Medical Journal* 46:181-186. PubMed Reference UI: 91188893.

Sierpina, V. S., B. Wollschlaeger, and M. Blumenthal. 2003. Ginkgo biloba. *American Family Physician Journal* (September 1).

Sobow, T., and I. Kloszewska. 2003. Donepezil plus vitamin E as a treatment in Alzheimer disease. *Alzheimer Disease & Associated Disorders Journal* 17(4):244.

Sparks, D. L., T. A. Martin, D. R. Gross, and J. C. Hunsaker III. 2000. Link between heart disease, cholesterol and Alzheimer's: A review. *Microscopy Research Technique* 50(4):287-290.

Sunderland, T., G. Linker, N. Mirza, K. T. Putnam, D. I. Friedman, L. H. Kimmel, et al. 2003. Decreased B-amyloid$_{1-42}$ and increased tau levels in cerebrospinal fluid of patients with Alzheimer's disease. *JAMA* 289:2094-2103.

Tanzi, R. E., and A. B. Parson. 2000. *Decoding Darkness: The Search for the Genetic Causes of Alzheimer's Disease.* Cambridge, MA: Perseus Publishing.

Vukovic, L. 1998. The best herbs for every stage of your life. *Natural Health Magazine* September/October, 1998.

Weil, A. 1998. *Eight Weeks to Optimum Health.* New York: Ballantine Books.

Werbach, M. R., 1993. *Nutritional Influences on Illness.* New York: Third Line Press, Inc.

Huang, X., P. Math, C. Cuajungco, C. S Atwood, R. D. Moir, R. E. Tanzi et al. 2000. Alzheimer's disease, ß-amyloid protein and zinc. *Journal of Nutrition* 130:1488(S)-1492(S).

Zandi, P., J. C. Anthony, A. S. Khachaturian, S. V. Stone, D. Gustavson, et al. 2004. Reduced risk of Alzheimer disease in users of antioxidant vitamin supplements: The Cache County Study. *JAMA Archives of Neurology* 61(1):82-88.

Zeisel, S. H., M. H. Mar, J. C. Howe, and J. M. Holden. 2003. Concentrations of choline-containing compounds and betaine in common foods. *Journal of Nutrition* 133:1302-1307.

Some Other
New Harbinger Titles

Solid to the Core, Item 4305 $14.95

Staying Focused in the Age of Distraction, Item 433X $16.95

Living Beyond Your Pain, Item 4097 $19.95

Fibromyalgia & Chronic Fatigue Syndrome, Item 4593 $14.95

Your Miraculous Back, Item 4526 $18.95

TriEnergetics, Item 4453 $15.95

Emotional Fitness for Couples, Item 4399 $14.95

The MS Workbook, Item 3902 $19.95

Depression & Your Thyroid, Item 4062 $15.95

The Eating Wisely for Hormonal Balance Journal, Item 3945 $15.95

Healing Adult Acne, Item 4151 $15.95

The Memory Doctor, Item 3708 $11.95

The Emotional Wellness Way to Cardiac Health, Item 3740 $16.95

The Cyclothymia Workbook, Item 383X $18.95

The Matrix Repatterning Program for Pain Relief, Item 3910 $18.95

Transforming Stress, Item 397X $10.95

Eating Mindfully, Item 3503 $13.95

Living with RSDS, Item 3554 $16.95

The Ten Hidden Barriers to Weight Loss, Item 3244 $11.95

The Sjogren's Syndrome Survival Guide, Item 3562 $15.95

Stop Feeling Tired, Item 3139 $14.95

Responsible Drinking, Item 2949 $19.95

The Mitral Valve Prolapse/Dysautonomia Survival Guide,
Item 3031 $14.95

The Vulvodynia Survival Guide, Item 2914 $16.95

Call **toll free, 1-800-748-6273,** or log on to our online bookstore at **www.newharbinger.com** to order. Have your Visa or Mastercard number ready. Or send a check for the titles you want to New Harbinger Publications, Inc., 5674 Shattuck Ave., Oakland, CA 94609. Include $4.50 for the first book and 75¢ for each additional book, to cover shipping and handling. (California residents please include appropriate sales tax.) Allow two to five weeks for delivery.

Prices subject to change without notice.